Advance Praise for *Knowledge to Action*

"In support of a critical effort to support a Culture of Health in America comes this comprehensive and expertly written and edited volume by a diverse group of experts. Sponsored by America's largest foundation devoted to health and well-being, it is a manifesto that explains a Culture of Health and presents a multi-faceted rationale and the ingredients required from multiple sectors of our economy. It also describes how to vet, choose, employ, and evaluate supportive policies, programs, and system changes to improve the health of individuals and communities. This seminal work should be required reading for all devoted to improving population health."
—**Jonathan Fielding, MD, MA, MPH, MBA, Distinguished Professor, UCLA Fielding Schools of Public Health and Geffen School of Medicine, and Founder and Co-Director, the UCLA Center for Health Advancement**

"The Robert Wood Johnson Foundation's *Knowledge to Action* volume is essential reading for those grappling with the most important health issues in the nation. While making it clear there are no easy answers, it entertainingly illuminates what we know and don't know about such topics as health equity, climate change, and violence. Simply hearing from some of the country's wisest voices and most innovative researchers is worth the read. But the book goes farther and shows us multiple pathways to improving the health and well-being of the nation's residents, some of them already being taken with support from the Foundation and others."
—**John Auerbach, MBA, President and CEO, Trust for America's Health**

"Achieving a society which ensures that everyone has an equal opportunity to live a long life of high quality is an important national goal. However, achieving such a culture requires identifying best practices and building the collaborative systems to ensure success. This publication, the first in a series, is a practical look into how we see culture and covers key concepts on how to make health a shared vision and innovative ways to build systems to achieve it. It is a timely and practical resource for those on the quest to achieve a Culture of Health."
—**Georges Benjamin, MD, Executive Director, American Public Health Association**

"*Knowledge to Action* addresses the wicked problem of how do we in the United States achieve a Culture of Health that becomes part of the "taken for granted" way of being an American? A wicked problem is one in which we do not even know what we do not know. This edited volume pushes back the veil of ignorance with both humility and audacity. A diverse mix of "thinking doers" and "doing thinkers" share their knowledge and experience creating a major step toward making the Culture of Health Action Framework come alive. It highlights the need for not only expanding opportunities for cross-sector collaboration but expanding the number of people with access to those opportunities and their benefits that have historically been denied. *Knowledge to Action* will produce a spark to take action in all who read it."

—Stephen M. Shortell, PhD, MPH, MBA, Blue Cross of California Distinguished Professor of Health Policy and Management and Dean Emeritus, School of Public Health, University of California, Berkeley

"The outstanding contributors and the artful editing by Dr. Alonzo Plough make *Knowledge to Action* a persuasive and usable tool for everyone from academic teachers to public health practitioners. The vivid examples, personal perspectives and compelling data in this book highlight why a new Culture of Health is needed."

—Paul K. Halverson, DrPH, MHSA, FACHE, Founding Dean and Professor, Richard M. Fairbanks School of Public Health, Indiana University

"*Knowledge to Action* is a welcome contribution to efforts for equity in health and its determinants. It will be a compelling read for those who work to produce knowledge that has a decent chance of leading to action for greater health equity, and for those laboring in the trenches, directly engaged in action for greater health equity, who want their actions to be informed by the best available knowledge. The editors have identified many important, challenging issues and assembled an impressive and thoughtful panel of authors who have the expertise to go beneath the surface in addressing those issues."

—Paula Braveman, MD, MPH, Professor, University of California, San Francisco

"The Robert Wood Johnson Foundation has changed the conversation about health in the United States. This important volume further advances the understanding of factors in our society that must be aligned to create the healthy living environments and healthy choices needed for individual and community health and to achieving the treatment and prevention goals of the medical care system. The United States is now an urban nation and chapters on the creation of healthy cities stimulate an important future discussion as do models of social investment needed to bring important private capital into partnerships with government to achieve a Culture of Health in our nation."

—Jo Ivey Boufford, MD, President, The New York Academy of Medicine

Knowledge to Action

Knowledge to Action

Accelerating Progress in Health, Well-Being, and Equity

EDITED BY ALONZO L. PLOUGH, PHD, MPH, MA

OXFORD
UNIVERSITY PRESS

OXFORD
UNIVERSITY PRESS

Oxford University Press is a department of the University of Oxford. It furthers
the University's objective of excellence in research, scholarship, and education
by publishing worldwide. Oxford is a registered trade mark of Oxford University
Press in the UK and certain other countries.

Published in the United States of America by Oxford University Press
198 Madison Avenue, New York, NY 10016, United States of America.

Library of Congress Cataloging-in-Publication Data
Names: Sharing Knowledge to Build a Culture
of Health Conference (2016 :Baltimore, Md.), author. | Plough, Alonzo L., editor.
Title: Knowledge to action : accelerating progress in health, well-being,
and equity / [edited by] Alonzo Louis Plough.
Description: Oxford ; New York : Oxford University Press, [2017] | Includes
bibliographical references and index.
Identifiers: LCCN 2017000265 (print) | LCCN 2017001443 (ebook) |
ISBN 9780190669348 (pbk. : alk. paper) |
ISBN 9780190669355 (UPDF) | ISBN 9780190669362 (EPUB)
Subjects: | MESH: Health Equity | Public Health | Health Promotion |
Attitude to Health | United States | Congresses
Classification: LCC RA427 (print) | LCC RA427 (ebook) | NLM W 76 AA1 |
DDC 362.1—dc23
LC record available at https://lccn.loc.gov/2017000265

3 5 7 9 8 6 4 2
Printed by Sheridan Books, Inc., United States of America

CONTENTS

PREFACE

ALONZO L. PLOUGH, PHD, MPH, MA, CHIEF SCIENCE OFFICER
AND VICE PRESIDENT, RESEARCH-EVALUATION-LEARNING,
ROBERT WOOD JOHNSON FOUNDATION

This is the inaugural volume of a publication series from the Robert Wood Johnson Foundation (RWJF) that we hope will catalyze discussion, engage new partners, and inspire action to build a Culture of Health in America. The content and approach of the series reflect the movement from RWJF's previous vision statement and the preceding publication series, titled "To Improve Health and Heath Care," to our current call to action for ourselves and the nation to build a Culture of Health—where all individuals, organizations, communities, and sectors value health as a shared goal and work together to improve well-being. This is a bolder goal that requires us all to think and work differently, and to incorporate diverse perspectives, innovative sources of knowledge, and practical experiences from those who are in the agencies, organizations, and community coalitions working in their own way to improve population health, well-being, and equity.

This volume is a lively and accessible edited version of our inaugural *Sharing Knowledge to Build a Culture of Health* conference, held in March 2016 in Baltimore, Md. Nearly 400 researchers, practitioners, and policymakers representing multiple sectors and diverse viewpoints gathered to engage in an exciting exchange of ideas around the critical assessment, challenges, and innovative thinking required to reach the goal of building a Culture of Health. While distinguished researchers from many different fields were contributors and attendees, the conference was organized around highlighting actionable knowledge from a variety of sources that skewed more practical than purely academic in orientation. Exploring a variety of rigorous approaches to evidence that include, but extend beyond, conventional approaches to health and health care research is a theme that runs through the ideas presented in this volume. Chapter contributors include journalists, writers, planners, architects, and community activists. Topics range from Ta-Nehisi Coates's exploration of the pervasiveness of fear that shaped his experience of inequity as a youth in Baltimore, to Steven Woolf's explication of the use of big data analytics to support public health and social policy decision-making in San Diego. What ties all of the presentations and discussions together is a focus on how different levels of information—including on-the-ground experience, data and methodology, collaboration strategies, and policy analysis—can be integrated to improve our efforts to build a Culture of Health.

Each chapter that follows combines the formal presentations, audience questions, and additional insights and conversations among the session panel participants on the stated topics. The chapters have been edited to present the different perspectives of the presenters, the energetic dialogue that the presentations elicited, and how this informs a general set of issues directly related to the Culture of Health vision and Action Framework. Some of the presentations represent projects funded by RWJF. Others represent innovative research and ideas that are relevant to RWJF's work, but have been developed without our funding. There are framing introductions to each section that connect them to the larger issues in the field and future knowledge building and action challenges.

The volume proceeds as follows:

Section 1, an introduction by Risa Lavizzo-Mourey, presents a general overview of how RWJF developed the Culture of Health vision and Action Framework and her personal reflections on the important roles the conference and this new publication series play in advancing RWJF's overall strategy.

Section 2, *Views on Understanding Culture, Experience, and Health*, includes the dynamic keynote session of the conference, highlighting the presentations of Ta-Nehisi Coates on contexts of fear in urban America and Anne Case on the conditions of despair in largely rural America that create health inequity. It continues with excerpts from David R. Williams' powerful presentation on how we must move from disparity to equity. The section concludes with the integration of three presentations using survey research approaches to understand how Americans value (or don't value) health by Larry Bye, Dante Chinni, and Alia Crum.

Section 3, *Pursuing Knowledge with Purpose*, begins with five insightful viewpoints on how to better understand that the methods we use to develop evidence are themselves subject to certain assumptions and even biases, which influence policy and decision-making processes. Under the provocative chapter title *The Tyranny of Evidence*, Karen Pittman, Lisbeth Schorr,

Rajiv Mehta, Emily E. Tanner-Smith, and Brian S. Mittman explore the question of what kinds of evidence tell us "what works" in the context of building a Culture of Health. The chapter *Measure the Change You Wish to See in the World* follows. Karen Matsuoka, Carly Riley, Sarah Burd-Sharps, and Bruce Y. Lee investigate how we define well-being in a society and how can we measure it and track changes over time. Next, in the chapter *The Secrecy Divide: Sharing Data Across Sectors*, Heather Joseph, Joshua M. Sharfstein, and Steven H. Woolf address the challenging issue of sharing information across governmental-, academic-, and community-level data generators and users to better understand the social determinants of health. In the final chapter, *The Importance of Community-Based Participatory Research*, Christopher Gibbons and Consuelo H. Wilkins discuss the importance of deep community collaboration and engagement in research and the challenges both in academia and in communities to achieve successful partnerships.

Section 4, *Critical Pathways for Systems Change*, explores how building a Culture of Health requires a special focus on understanding and improving the systems and environments that are most significant to improving well-being. The first chapter, *Fostering Healthier Environments for Children and Families*, addresses the critical question of what must be done to strengthen families and ensure that children are heathy and thriving throughout their life course. The contributors, representing a wide range of perspectives, are Debra L. Ness, Ron Haskins, Max Crowley, and Eboni Howard. The next chapter takes on the major issue of *Aligning Systems of Health and Health Care*, which is an action area of the Culture of Health Action Framework and perhaps the focal health policy issue for our nation. What are the innovations that will re-balance our $3 trillion health care expenditures toward investments in prevention and community and social resources? Contributors are Sherry Glied, Manik Bhat, Manmeet Kaur, and Rocco Perla. Next, *Building Healthy Cities*, focuses on the fact that 80 percent of the U.S. population lives in metropolitan areas and urbanization will be the key demographic force over the next 45 years. How will our cities accommodate physical activity, open space, and equitable planning and design? Gil Penalosa, Kate DeSantis, and Ela Rausch address these questions. The next chapter addresses a major crisis facing our nation: *Rethinking How We Police Communities*. The collective trauma resulting from conflict and mistrust between law enforcement and the communities they protect has not been successfully addressed from either the health or the criminal justice systems. Auke van Dijk, Amanda Geller, and John Rich provide different perspectives and insights on this important problem. The final chapter addresses the largest influence on our health and well-being globally, as defined by the World Health Organization (WHO): *Climate Change Through a Health Lens.* Climate change is most often thought of as an environmental matter, but the real consequences on health and health disparities are already evident and measurable. Linda Rudolph, Sabrina McCormick, and Eric Klinenberg provide their diverse perspectives on this critical issue.

Section 5, *Innovating to Build a Culture of Health,* presents different approaches to catalyzing innovation across sectors and disciplines to build a Culture of Health. In the first chapter, *Public, Private, Nonprofit Partnership: A Case Study of Social Impact Bonds,* Andrea Phillips, Chris Ellis, and John Roman describe a new approach to using private investment dollars to provide capital incentives to improve health and human services impacts. The next chapter, *Forward in Baltimore: Illuminating the Possible, Achieving the Potential,* featuring Leana S. Wen and Lew Daly, moves from the market incentive orientation of the previous chapter to focus on innovation that intergovernmental coordination and community partnerships can achieve. In the final chapter, *A Look Inside the Robert Wood Johnson Foundation,* Priya Gandhi and Brian C. Quinn describe how RWJF is working in both traditional and new areas across diverse sectors to accelerate progress toward building a Culture of Health.

ACKNOWLEDGMENTS

ALONZO L. PLOUGH, PHD, MPH, MA, CHIEF SCIENCE OFFICER
AND VICE PRESIDENT, RESEARCH-EVALUATION-LEARNING,
ROBERT WOOD JOHNSON FOUNDATION

Planning the inaugural *Sharing Knowledge to Build a Culture of Health* conference involved many individuals, both internal and external to RWJF. I want to thank Lisa Simpson, MB, BCh, MPH, FAAP, and her staff at AcademyHealth for collaborating with us to convene this conference, and the external scientific advisory group who helped develop the panel topics and identified speakers. At RWJF, Priya Gandhi, MS, managed our support of the conference and the coordination with AcademyHealth. Brian C. Quinn, PhD, provided sage leadership throughout the planning process.

Turning an exciting and idea-packed three-day conference into a book also required the vision and support of many. The Editorial Review Group has oversight of the development of this series, and provided careful commentary and suggestions for this volume. My colleagues in this group are:

Sandro Galea, MD, MPH, DPH, Boston University
Sherry Glied, PhD, MA, New York University
Frederick Mann, Robert Wood Johnson Foundation
James Marks, MD, MPH, Robert Wood Johnson Foundation
Chad Zimmerman, Oxford University Press

A team within RWJF worked on a tight timeline to produce the manuscript with Gandhi's able operations management. Additional thanks to:

Tanya Barrientos
Ed Ghisu, JD
Sofia Kounelias
Risa Lavizzo-Mourey, MD, MBA
Brian C. Quinn, PhD
Kristin Silvani

Finally, a talented team of editorial consultants produced wonderfully integrated drafts from the original presentations. They are:

Karyn Feiden
Mary B. Geisz, PhD
Karen Gross
Margaret O. Kirk
Mary Nakashian, MS

PART ONE

INTRODUCTION

Accelerating a Culture of Health by Sharing Knowledge and Acting Together

RISA LAVIZZO-MOUREY, MD, MBA, PRESIDENT AND CEO,
ROBERT WOOD JOHNSON FOUNDATION

On March 9, 2016, the Robert Wood Johnson Foundation (RWJF) welcomed a capacity crowd to the inaugural *Sharing Knowledge to Build a Culture of Health* conference, which you'll read about on the pages to follow.

This was not a convening of like-minded, longstanding allies. Distinguished researchers, practitioners, and policymakers gathered in Baltimore from across various sectors. Many were meeting for the first time. And together, we began to write a new chapter in the national effort to improve health—a chapter highlighted by cross-sector collaboration and action.

How did we get here?

In 2014, RWJF announced a new vision to build a Culture of Health in America—a culture that values health as the bedrock of personal fulfillment and the backbone of a strong, competitive nation. I described our discovery of the Culture of Health vision in the previous iteration of this series, *To Improve Health and Health Care, Volume XVI*, which we published in 2015. In essence, we ascertained that health is everything—linked to health care, yet extending to the grander whole of work, family, and community life. We envisioned a society where the healthy choice is the easy choice for all.

We knew from the get-go that RWJF couldn't possibly build a Culture of Health alone—nor should we. This vision calls for us, as a nation, *to strive together to build a Culture of Health enabling all in our diverse society to lead healthier lives, now and for generations to come.* It invites us to think big and take bold steps with others, because the need for improved health and well-being is urgent.

Even though we spend far more on health than other developed countries, Americans live sicker, shorter lives. And while we say that our kids are our future, there is a very real chance that this generation may be the first to live sicker and die younger than their parents' generation. Did you know, for example, that more than 70 percent of young adults in the United States would not qualify for military service because they are too obese, too poorly educated, or too tangled up in drugs or crime?[1]

The *Sharing Knowledge* conference brought together bright minds across disciplines to think about and tackle such multipronged challenges. Academics participated alongside architects. Experts in early childhood and families conversed with innovators in community development and finance. Thought-leaders in public health networked with pioneers in policing and climate change. There was palpable electricity in the air, sparked by the promise of unique perspectives, unconventional collaborations, and unlimited possibilities.

With this book, we aimed to bottle some of that lightning.

For a Culture of Health to take root, it has to be cultivated by those who have not historically seen themselves as influencers of health and well-being.

Why? Because our health is inextricably tied to where we live, learn, work, and play. We cannot expect the health sector to address all of these factors singlehandedly. Changing the trajectory of America's health requires joining forces.

RWJF has long been known for our ability to convene and create alliances between "strange bedfellows." In fact, during our fledgling years in the early 1970s, we brought an unlikely coalition of policy wonks, physicians, police and fire departments, and ambulance services together to catalyze the national 911 emergency call system.

In that spirit, we have over the past three years intentionally disrupted the echo chamber of our own thinking by expanding our network, invigorating existing relationships, and helping others make new connections. To build a comprehensive Culture of Health, we've started to work differently both internally and with others, with an eye toward being more adaptable, action-oriented, and collaborative. We are fostering the institutional courage to forge uncharted paths and unexpected partnerships over the long term.

In late 2015, we unveiled an **Action Framework** to guide our efforts and those of the nation.[2] Rigorously developed in collaboration with the RAND

---

[1] Source: 2016 Citizen-Readiness Index, available at *www.strongnation.org.*

[2] The Culture of Health Action Framework was released in the report *From Vision to Action: A Framework and Measures to Mobilize a Culture of Health,* which can be downloaded at *www.cultureofhealth.org.*

Corporation, and with key input from more than 1,000 experts, partners, global leaders, and others, the Framework is intended to mobilize the Culture of Health vision and measure our nation's progress. It builds on the legacy of those who have advanced innovation and collaboration in the health arena for years. And it is meant to invite *new* participants by helping them see the transformative roles they can play, or may already be playing, to improve health for all.

The Framework is grounded in four interconnected Action Areas, designed to catalyze more integrated collaborations:

1. **Making Health a Shared Value**

    This Action Area puts our nation's goals about better health front and center. When we do that, we will be able to fuel an increased demand for healthy places and practices, a greater sense of community, and a stronger belief that individual actions can make a difference in the well-being of others.

2. **Fostering Cross-Sector Collaboration to Improve Well-Being**

    This Action Area highlights the importance of collaborations that include sectors typically considered outside the realm of health care, such as business, law enforcement, transportation, education, and environmental organizations.

3. **Creating Healthier, More Equitable Communities**

    Not all places give people the opportunity to make healthy choices. The goal of this Action Area is to improve the communities where people live, learn, work, and play, so everyone has a fair chance to thrive.

4. **Strengthening Integration of Health Services and Systems**

    This Action Area encourages better balance and integration between medical treatment, public health, and social services. It represents RWJF's long-standing and ongoing commitment to improving health and health care in America.

Each of these Action Areas includes a set of **Drivers**—long-term priorities that individuals and organizations across sectors can focus on to accelerate progress in health, both nationally and at the community level. (For instance, the Drivers in Action Area 1 include Mind-set and Expectations, Sense of Community, and Civic Engagement.) Together, the Action Areas and the Drivers create the key building blocks of the Action Framework that will remain constant over time.

The Framework also includes national, evidence-based **Measures**, selected as points of assessment and engagement. The Measures are not limited to traditional health indicators; instead, they encourage us to think about and gauge health in broader ways, incorporating all aspects of well-being. To explore the

Action Areas, Drivers, and Measures in detail, and to draw inspiration from real-world examples, I encourage you to visit *www.cultureofhealth.org*.

The Action Framework will guide all facets of RWJF's work over the next 20 years: from the issues we focus on, to our investments, to how we approach program development and evaluation. And while we plan to fund work in all four of the Action Areas, we will not cover every aspect of the four. We recognize that RWJF is one of many organizations working toward the common cause of improving health in America. The Framework was designed to provide numerous entry points for involvement, and to inspire many individuals, communities, and sectors to build a Culture of Health in their own unique ways.

When we make progress in these four integrated Action Areas, we believe the nation will significantly improve overall population health, well-being, and equity. I'd like to emphasize the importance of equity not only as an intended outcome but also as an overarching theme—deeply infused into the entire Action Framework, and a key through line of the *Sharing Knowledge* conference.

Health equity means working together to make sure that we *all* have the basics to be healthy. Personal responsibility and behavior play a key role in health. But the choices we make depend on the opportunities we have available to us.

RWJF is focused on building a Culture of Health where everyone has a fair chance to live a healthier life. Across the country, communities are finding creative solutions. We want to work with them, learn from them, and share what works. Because highlighting the inequities we face is not enough. We must take action.

We realize that achieving health equity may require candid and, at times, challenging conversations about race, violence, poverty, and other contentious issues. We did not shy away from discussing such sensitive topics at the *Sharing Knowledge* conference or in this book. We acknowledge the complexity of these issues and the wide range of perspectives they elicit.

During the conference's keynote plenary, entitled *Achieving Equity*, I explored some of these very issues along with Dr. Anne Case and Ta-Nehisi Coates, both influential thought-leaders whose work has provoked widespread conversation and media coverage. As you'll read in the first chapter, Case's academic study illuminates a sharp increase in the death rate for middle-aged whites after 1998, which she describes as an overlooked epidemic of "deaths of despair." Coates' narrative combines extensive research with personal experience to describe the impact of inequity and fear on the black body.

Case and Coates have distinct approaches to generating and sharing knowledge. Yet, taken together, their work suggests how we—as generators and users of knowledge—might employ research *and* narrative to communicate effectively about health equity. And, as we build a Culture of Health, we must consider how we can do a better job of making data more widely accessible and embracing a diversity of stories so everyone can find their place in the movement.

How does research translate into conversation, collaboration, and action? Are there new approaches and applications we might consider?

As I mulled over these questions throughout the conference, I was struck by Dr. John Rich's thinking about the pathway from knowledge to action, discussed later in this book, in *Rethinking How We Police Communities.*

Rich is a professor in the Dornsife School of Public Health at Drexel University, where he also co-directs the Center for Nonviolence and Social Justice. His work focuses on black men in urban settings, and he received a 2006 MacArthur Foundation Fellowship for designing "new models of health care that stretch across the boundaries of public health, education, social service, and justice systems to engage young men in caring for themselves and their peers."

In approaching his work, Rich has utilized the three pillars of "Looking, Understanding, and Making"—a design construct inspired by Bill Lucas of the LUMA Institute in Pittsburgh. Applying this construct to research, Rich interprets "Looking" as data gathering; "Understanding" as data analysis; and "Making" as not only producing research, but creating and testing new solutions to wicked problems.

I recognized the parallels between this process of "Looking, Understanding, and Making" and RWJF's concentration on embracing the practices of emergent strategy to build a Culture of Health. As we become more purposeful about embedding these ideas into our work, and encouraging others to move from knowledge to action, "Looking, Understanding, and Making" strikes me as a user-friendly approach.

For instance, I find Case's work to be a good example of the "Understanding" pillar and the ongoing need to evaluate how information is interpreted and presented. After all, she and co-researcher Sir Angus Deaton discovered the troubling mortality trend while analyzing an existing data set.

In his presentation, Rich shared the following quote from the human-centered design consultant Lucas Nene: "If you are looking and understanding, but not making, then you are really just daydreaming." These words remind us that we must maintain an unwavering commitment to reaching the stage of action, where progress happens.

We are heartened to see how the Culture of Health vision and Action Framework are encouraging people across the nation to join forces and act together to improve health, well-being, and equity. In RWJF's 2016 Annual Message, I pointed to specific organizations that are connecting with the Action Framework, establishing unexpected partnerships, and reaping extraordinary results.

For example, Spartanburg Regional Healthcare System in South Carolina formed a partnership with 10 community organizations to create AccessHealth Spartanburg, designed to connect low-income, uninsured people to health care and address barriers to health services. By better coordinating primary care and focusing on the social issues that affect health—such as transportation, access to medications, housing, and employment—the program reduced hospital costs for the targeted population by 42 percent and hospital admissions by 31 percent.

Building a Culture of Health is a long-term proposition, requiring the involvement and investment of many. To sustain the movement, and especially to improve equity, we must listen to how others define health and embrace different perspectives. We must join together in purpose and accountability. And we must remain focused on providing a healthier future for our children.

I would be remiss if I didn't recognize those who ushered the *Sharing Knowledge to Build a Culture of Health* conference from vision to reality. Dr. Alonzo L. Plough, RWJF's Vice President for Research-Evaluation-Learning and Chief Science Officer, and many others from RWJF worked tirelessly to orchestrate an unprecedented meeting of the minds in Baltimore. Dr. Lisa Simpson and the team from AcademyHealth were excellent collaborators, making the conference run smoothly and successfully. The external scientific advisory group was instrumental in identifying a robust and engaging lineup of topics and speakers. And, of course, I'm truly grateful for the distinguished speakers who shared their knowledge at the conference and in this book.

As I conclude my tenure as RWJF's president and CEO, I couldn't be more proud to launch *The Culture of Health Series*, starting with this volume. Inspired by the Culture of Health vision, these publications are intended to be vital, valuable, and topical resources for the work of improving health. My hope is that you—the person who has picked up this book—will put what you learn into action.

It has been a great privilege to help advance the vision of building a Culture of Health in America. I look forward to watching that vision continue to blossom.

PART TWO

VIEWS ON UNDERSTANDING CULTURE, EXPERIENCE, AND HEALTH

Views on Understanding Culture, Experience, and Health highlights the deep divide that separates Americans from one another. In neighborhoods and communities across the country, and especially where underserved and underrepresented populations live, learn, work, and play, multiple layers of discrimination, segregation, lack of mobility, and inadequate public policies are fueling pain and anguish. The stories of the people who live this reality are an urgent reminder that failing to act on long-standing social issues is perpetuating a crisis in health and well-being.

The three chapters in this section illustrate how deeply disconnected some communities are from the structures of society that should support, not harm, them. The contributors—who represent diverse professions in economics, sociology, public health, policy and behavioral research, psychology, and journalism—combine research and personal narratives to explain what is at stake as they implore us to move from inequity to equity.

In *Fear and Despair: Consequences of Inequity* we are reminded of the harms done to the physical, emotional, and intellectual health of black children when communities are left behind, and learn, with the starkness of data, about a silent epidemic of diseases and deaths of despair afflicting middle-aged whites without college degrees.

From Disparity to Equity further highlights the racial inequalities that encroach on virtually every dimension of life, from housing to health care to wealth accumulation, as well as less-familiar indignities, such as the ability to hail a cab, earn a promotion, purchase insurance—or simply walk down the street without encountering discourtesy.

How Americans Value Health confronts the reality of our deeply divided society, where people still define health as an absence of illness, rather than putting health at the center of their lives.

The authors do not mince words. *The stakes could not be higher . . . There can be no Culture of Health until the American people develop greater awareness of these problems . . . American adults are highly divided in their health beliefs . . .* But they also offer a sense of possibility. In these chapters, the authors present compelling data and solutions to begin the critical movement from stark inequity toward a more equitable society. *We need ripples of hope,* they conclude. And that starts by both acknowledging the view from the ground up and embracing the value of the collective good embedded in a Culture of Health.

Fear and Despair

Consequences of Inequity

ANNE CASE, PHD, MPA, ALEXANDER STEWART 1886 PROFESSOR
OF ECONOMICS AND PUBLIC AFFAIRS, AND DIRECTOR, RESEARCH
PROGRAM IN DEVELOPMENT STUDIES, PRINCETON UNIVERSITY

TA-NEHISI COATES, NATIONAL CORRESPONDENT, *THE ATLANTIC*,
AND AUTHOR, *BETWEEN THE WORLD AND ME*

Given that equity is at once an intended outcome and an overarching theme of the Culture of Health, as Lavizzo-Mourey noted in her introduction, data and anecdote both have roles to play in deepening our understanding. With their stark portraits of the fear and despair that take over when equity is absent, Ta-Nehisi Coates and Anne Case make distinct and compelling arguments for attending to equity now.

Coates offered a powerful personal narrative to recreate the fears of a black child who comes to realize that his personal safety is always at risk and that he is on his own—the helping institutions protect some people from harm, but he is not among them.

Case's provocative analysis points to alarming increases in "diseases and deaths of despair" among middle-aged white adults. Believing that life will not improve for them, their mortality rates are rising, reflecting drug overdoses, suicide, and deaths from alcohol abuse.

Fear

There was a dawning awareness of the world in which we lived. And that world was violent. And that world was a world where our bodies could be threatened, where things could be done to us, and we couldn't depend on any sort of authority figure, any sort of force within society to protect us. Our personal safety was up to us.—Ta-Nehisi Coates

Through the lens of formative events in his youth, Ta-Nehisi Coates examined the lived experience of black children growing up in fear for their physical safety. His stories serve as commentary on the profound inequity that ensues when rules and institutions protect some children and abandon others. "I can't help but differentiate between the kind of environment that I grew up in—in Baltimore City—and the kind of environments I have been exposed to as an adult and that I see other children growing up in," he said.

School Days

What happens when the state retreats from its responsibility to protect the bodies of certain people and leaves it up to them to do that for themselves? And what happens when that is not true across the society, but is true only for certain communities?—Ta-Nehisi Coates

While visiting an upscale school in Washington, D.C., Coates was struck by the "lack of physical angst amongst the kids, or what appeared to me as a complete sense of physical safety, a cheerful go-luckiness that I certainly did not associate with going to school when I was a kid in Baltimore."

The warm atmosphere of learning in this school evoked in Coates a quite different experience, one of deploying his youthful energy and brainpower to securing his physical safety:

When I woke up in the morning, I wasn't thinking about whether I had finished my homework. I wasn't thinking about whether I had my assignments in order. I wasn't thinking about playing basketball after school.

I was thinking about how I was going to dress. I was thinking about how I was going to cock my hat, whether I was going to wear a hat or not. I was thinking about which jacket I was going to wear, what colors were going to be on that jacket. I was thinking about how I was going to carry my book bag. I was thinking about how many young boys I was going to walk to school with. I was thinking about where those young boys were from. I was thinking about what path we were going to take to school.

And once I got to school, I was thinking about who I had problems with in my classroom. I was thinking about where I was going to sit during lunchtime, whether I was going to go to lunch at all.

And then after school, I was thinking about when I was going to leave school, at what point and at what time. Who was going to be walking with me, where were they from, which path we were going to take home? And at every single instance, each of those decisions revolved around my attempt to secure the safety of my body.

Nights Out in the City

And there were no police and there were no adults. There was really just no anything.—Ta-Nehisi Coates

At 9:00 one summer night, nine-year-old Coates saw a group of boys coming toward him and his older brother as they waited for their ride home after attending a wrestling match. "It never occurred to me that they would do any sort of violence to us, but one of them punched my brother in the face. My brother takes off running, immediately grasping the situation."

Coates was "cut off by another young man, who punched me in the face. Then they went and pursued my brother and jumped my brother. And I stood under the awning of Lexington Market in Baltimore . . . and I can see this just as though it was yesterday, waves of young black boys coming down the street, jumping and beating on whoever might be unlucky enough to go past."

The lesson he drew from that experience: "I was ultimately accountable for my own protection; I was ultimately accountable for my own physical health."

That summer, Coates's 13-year-old brother bought a gun. "It was not so much that I knew that my brother had a gun that is extraordinary, but the fact that knowing that he had a gun was an un-extraordinary fact to me."

Policy Decisions Are Health Decisions

Even as I looked at people who I thought were rough and tough and had the ability to protect their bodies, to ensure their physical health, as anybody who works with data and looks at the kind of communities that I grew up in will show you, these efforts ultimately don't protect our bodies at all. It just looks like it.—Ta-Nehisi Coates

Coates's stories brought home the "physicality of racism"—its impact on the body and its impact on poor outcomes and inequitable outcomes for whole groups of people. Policies that tolerate attacks on young children, turn a blind eye to dangerous neighborhoods, fail to provide basic protection, and offer incarceration as an acceptable solution are all policies that influence health.

Conversations about race are filled with words—some call them euphemisms—that aim to describe the impact of racism on people and communities, Coates said. Ideas about affirmative action, job discrimination, housing discrimination, and racial justice all cycle back to "the physicality of racism, the impact on the actual body. Inequity in health is ultimately what you are talking about."

"When you talk about how the young boys that I grew up around walked through the world, when you talk about the fact that my brother had made a decision at 13–14 years old that he was going to carry a handgun, when you talk about the fact that that wasn't even unusual, you are talking about the physical safety, the danger, the very health of the body."

Despair

This is a story about a silent epidemic.—Anne Case

Anne Case used numbers to tell a story about poor health and early death among middle-aged whites. She presented findings from her comprehensive study of mortality and morbidity in the United States between 1998 and 2013.

An Unprecedented Rise in Mortality Among Middle-Aged Americans

For much of the 20th century, middle-aged Americans and citizens of other wealthy industrial countries enjoyed improved health and longer lives. Their mortality rates were falling steadily at the rate of about 2 percent per year.

Starting in about 1998, however, all-cause mortality among Americans ages 45 to 54 began to increase sharply, an "unprecedented" trend. Notably, mortality rates among people living in other wealthy countries continued to drop through this period.

While conducting a separate study of mortality rates and levels of general health, Anne Case and her colleague, Nobel laureate Sir Angus Deaton, PhD, noticed some disturbing patterns of deaths and illnesses and took a deeper look at their data[1] to find out what was happening.

But Not Among All Middle-Aged Americans

The answers surprised them. Mortality among middle-aged people was not rising across the board—there was an alarming year-by-year increase in mortality among white non-Hispanics ages 45 to 54 with high school degrees or less. The mortality rate for this group increased by 134 deaths per 100,000 people from 1999 to 2014.

This was not the case with middle-aged blacks or Hispanics. The mortality rate for middle-aged blacks (581 per 100,000 people) remained significantly

---

[1] Data sources for the study are the Centers for Disease Control and Prevention Wonder Compressed and Detailed Mortality files, individual death records, the American Community Surveys, the Current Population Surveys, and the Human Mortality Database.

higher than the middle-aged white rate (415 per 100,000 people) but continued to drop at about 2.6 percent per year. Middle-aged blacks "have been experiencing declines in mortality in middle age at a clip that is actually higher than those of the European comparison countries," notes Case.

The mortality rate for middle-aged Hispanic-Americans, at 262 per 100,000 people, was lower yet, declining by about 1.8 percent per year.

While the gap between black and white mortality rates has narrowed, Case cautioned against misguided optimism, noting that part of that is due to the increase in mortality among whites. "We may not want to benchmark progress in U.S. black longevity against U.S. whites," she said.

"If white mortality had continued to decline, a half-million lives would have been saved. That is the same order of magnitude as all the lives that have been lost in the U.S. to AIDS."

Diseases and Deaths That Need Not Occur

Three conditions—suicide, alcohol-related liver diseases, and accidental or deliberate intent undetermined drug overdoses (called "poisonings" by the Centers for Disease Control and Prevention)—account for most of the increase. As Anne Case observes, "What's driving this up really are what we call diseases or deaths of despair. These are deaths that do not have to happen. These are people who are taking their lives, either slowly or quickly." Middle-aged whites are most affected, but there has been an unrelenting climb in these deaths among every five-year cohort, from age 30 up to people in their 60s. Mortality rates from these conditions rose in lockstep across the four Census regions of the country: Northeast, Midwest, South, and West. Meanwhile, mortality rates among blacks from the three conditions remained generally flat across the age cohorts.

Case also found mortality rates for middle-aged whites increased year by year for each cause. Between 1998 and 2013:

• Deaths from suicide rose from just over 15 per 100,000 people to just over 25 per 100,000 people.
• Deaths from chronic liver disease rose from just over 15 per 100,000 people to just over 20 per 100,000 people.
• Deaths from overdoses rose from fewer than 5 per 100,000 people to 30 per 100,000 people.

Mortality rates from these causes for middle-aged whites with a high school degree or less rose by 22 percent between 1998 and 2013, while rates among people with college degrees remained essentially flat or fell somewhat during this period. Among whites ages 50 to 54:

- Men with a high school degree or less saw their mortality rise from just under 100 to just over 175 per 100,000 men.
- Women with a high school degree or less saw their mortality rise from about 25 to about 100 per 100,000 women.

The cause of these increases is not fully understood. Worsening financial stability among people with no more than high school degrees is a possible contributor, but the dramatic increase in deaths from overdoses is especially concerning.

"Where do these deaths from poisonings come from? It is opiates, so that is heroin, and opioids, which we call heroin in a pill. The new heroin epidemic is much whiter. It is much more suburban and rural than the 1970s heroin epidemic."

Case noted that both the number of prescriptions written for painkillers and the number of deaths from prescription overdoses tripled between 2000 and 2010. The CDC reports that in 2010 there were enough prescriptions written for painkillers to medicate every adult American around the clock for a month. Case laments, "This is the proximate cause for what's going on. But why has it touched all of these lives? What's going on here?"

More Pain and Stress, Less Well-Being

People's physical health is worse, their mental health is worse, their pain levels are higher, and they are having more difficulty socializing. This is accompanied by suicide, drug overdose, and slow death through alcohol. What do we do with this?—Anne Case

To learn more about possible drivers of the rise in mortality, Case explored how white middle-aged Americans rate their health and well-being.[2] Do they experience a lot of pain? Do they suffer from mental distress? Do they feel less able to work or engage in activities of daily living?

Sadly, the answer to all of these questions across the four Census regions is "yes." "Throughout the country, we are seeing a decline in people's sense of their own health," said Case.

Significantly fewer middle-aged whites say their health is excellent or very good. In comparing data for cohorts from 1993 to 1995 through 2011 to 2013,

---

[2] Data used to examine self-reported morbidity come from the National Health Interview Surveys, the Behavioral Risk Factor Surveillance System, and the National Health and Nutrition Examination Surveys.

Case found that self-reports of good health declined among younger people and increased among older people:

- In 2013, 55 percent of 50-year-olds said they were in excellent or very good health, down from 65 percent who reported excellent or very good health in 1995.
- In 2013, about 38 percent of 80-year-olds said they were in excellent or very good health, up from about 33 percent who reported excellent or very good health in 1995.

Case noted that these figures give the impression that there is a trade-off between young and old, making "health a zero-sum game. And we don't think it is a zero-sum game."

Middle-aged whites, unlike the young and the elderly, report more mental distress and chronic pain and more limitations in their ability to socialize, work, and conduct activities of daily living. Some significant changes reported between the years 1997 to 2000 and 2011 to 2014:

- Higher scores on a scale measuring serious mental distress.
- More reports of sciatica or joint pain, neck pain, and facial pain. By 2013, one in seven respondents said they had sciatica and one in three reported chronic joint pain.
- More reports of difficulty in socializing. "This one really troubles me," Case said, "as inability to socialize is a trigger for social isolation and for suicide."
- Reduced capacity to work. The fraction of people reporting inability to work doubled. By 2014, more than 10 percent of people in their 50s—prime working years—said they could not work.
- Significant deterioration in people's ability to walk a quarter mile, climb 10 steps, stand or sit for two hours, or shop.

Next Steps

Getting to deeper insights requires "getting into the weeds," said Case, "because we know all of these things affect all of the other things. Pain can affect mental health. Pain can also affect the amount of drugs you take, and drugs in turn can affect pain levels."

Questions she is exploring:

- Why is the United States different from European countries?
- Why is this a white phenomenon?
- Why does it affect both men and women?
- Are there some geographic areas that buck this trend and have lessons to offer?

Reflections

One group of Americans fears for their physical safety, suffers under practices that marginalize them, and struggles to thrive in environments that deny their experiences and dismiss their values. Another group, although benefitting from practices that promote their advancement and affirm their values, suffers from chronic debilitating physical and mental pain and untimely death.

Together, the story of fear and the study of despair call for deeper exploration of equity and compel the pursuit of common interests.

Equity: The Idea and the Reality

> When you have an ailing population, to what extent should we devote resources to changes in the health status of a population that is less ailing, that enjoys more privilege?—Ta-Nehisi Coates

In the discussions that followed the presentations, Camara Jones, MD, MPH, PhD, president of the American Public Health Association, sparked a heated conversation about equity by putting forth a challenge to the notion that a study focusing on middle-aged whites addresses equity.

"Achieving health equity requires at least three things: valuing all individuals and populations equally, recognizing and rectifying historical injustices, and providing resources according to need," Jones said.

White Americans have disproportionately benefitted from public policies and enjoy "the most privileged health status, even though there was a troubling change in their health status," she said. Jones maintained that "the crying need in our nation is not on that group," which, despite its challenges, has access to more resources and enjoys better health status than black Americans.

Jones asked Case why, when equity is the circle surrounding a Culture of Health, her presentation did not include more than just passing mention of the much-higher mortality rate among blacks.

Case explained that their findings emerged from a separate study originally intended to examine suicide in the United States. It was in the course of conducting that study that she observed that suicide among whites had increased and was more prevalent than among blacks.

Case fully agreed that equity is the core of a healthy society and is bothered by misleading reports that simply tout a shrinking gap between black and white mortality. While true, she warned that the shrinking gap comes partly from rising mortality among whites. "When we think about equity, we don't want to be thinking about leveling down. We want to think about bringing everybody to the frontier."

That raised the question of how best to redirect the entire research, investment, and policy enterprise at equity. "I think that's the question for this conference," said Lavizzo-Mourey, turning the challenge back to the audience. "We've got to create our own urgency and our own agenda for addressing the research, and also figure out how we're going to use this research to spark the kind of policy change that we need. It is not either/or. It is both/and."

Looking only at people with the poorest health is not likely to provide sufficient guidance, according to Case. Noting that mortality rates among Hispanic-Americans and Asian-Americans have steadily decreased at the same time mortality for whites has steadily increased, she suggested that probing differences among groups can answer some "why" questions: "Why is it that some groups are making a lot out of a little and some groups are not making much progress when they have such an abundance of resources?" Returning the conversation to Jones's challenging question about applying equity principles to health issues affecting whites, Coates articulated an uneasy reality. While acknowledging that increasing mortality in any group is troubling, he observed that the alarming declines in health uncovered in Case's research affected "the same people who would not want people like me moving next door."

Finding Common Ground

The fact that blacks are less likely than whites to receive prescriptions for opioid pain medications, and therefore are perhaps less apt to develop overdose problems, suggested to RWJF's Alonzo L. Plough a potential frame for common ground: "I think the question is around marginality—the shifting face of marginality that may affect different populations at different times. I would like to think about some of the commonalities around how we deal with marginalization." Coates expanded on Plough's thought: "We are observing something that is happening among a group that enjoys a level of privilege that people in the community I hail from do not enjoy. When you look at a community that has all the resources and yet you see their basic health outcomes declining, that tells you that there's something probably structurally wrong."

He suggested another area of common ground: both his and Case's presentations addressed the harm done to people's bodies, and notes that this harm follows from "big, broad policy decisions that had already been made . . . Problem neighborhoods exist because our country has made policy decisions. These are not mistakes," said Coates.

Coates called for a long-term investment to solve these long-term problems: "When we wanted to have negative outcomes in those communities, it is not like we practiced Jim Crow for a year. You know, we practiced it over a long period of time."

Divisiveness and Trust: Is Good Health a Zero-Sum Game?

> *I think one of the things we're trying to do in our country is understand how those divides are changing and what that implies for the kinds of conversations we hold. As far as trust, it's pretty elusive. It implies that we have meaningful conversations, to use research as a way of talking to one another and build that trust.* —Risa Lavizzo-Mourey

Gary Slutkin, MD, director of Cure Violence, added a dimension to the discussion prompted by Jones's opening question. He saw the divisiveness of the 2016 electoral process as a stark manifestation of the anger and frustration felt by many groups of Americans—blacks whose lives are devalued and whose children are traumatized, middle-aged whites who are getting sicker and dying younger, and others as well.

Eric Hekler, PhD, assistant professor at the School of Nutrition and Health Promotion at Arizona State University, introduced the role of *trust*, noting that RWJF's agenda for Culture of Health relies on a "basic building block of trust." He asked whether, given the depth of divisiveness, our country has the capacity to make progress, to develop that trust.

Coates ended by wondering whether people are invested in things besides living a longer life. "Are there things they want out of their lives that are worth something beyond whether their life span is actually increasing or declining? That is just a thought, just a question. I think we sometimes get too tied in with identifying groups of people's interests in a way that reflects our own interests."

Looking Abroad

Through much of history in the United States, a high school degree would secure a good job with benefits, on-the-job training, and opportunities for advancement, said Case. "Those jobs are gone. Those jobs aren't coming back."

Yet, other countries have lost jobs too, but their mortality rates continue to decline. "At what point did France see its jobs leave for Cambodia, at what point did the United Kingdom see its work being sent to Vietnam? What happened to those labor forces, to the people who got left behind? Somehow there is a whole population in those countries that is keeping body and soul together in a way that is not happening in the United States," said Case.

Coates agreed there are things to be learned from other places, but cautioned that sometimes "the things we really love about other places may be tied to things we don't actually like."

He struggled to reconcile the creation of a "broad and robust and strong social safety net without some corresponding definition of what it means to belong and to be part of society. And whenever people start doing that, they immediately start excluding other people."

> *I am not confident that conversations change because people acquire knowledge or willpower or are spiritually moved. I think conversations often change because a previous conversation becomes too expensive and unsupportable.*—Ta-Nehisi Coates

Black children and white adults usually live quite different lives. But, as Coates and Case so powerfully demonstrated, both are hurting. Why does a country with so many resources and so much talent tolerate the inequities that allow millions of people to live in fear and millions more to live in despair?

Ultimately, political decisions drive the answers and changing those decisions requires a shift in how we talk about them.

Achieving equity is difficult, but it is simply not an option to say it is impossible. The stories told by Coates and Case were about real people, people who are our relatives, neighbors, and colleagues. Our well-being and our future are intertwined with theirs. The stakes couldn't be higher.

From Disparity to Equity

DAVID R. WILLIAMS, PHD, MPH, FLORENCE SPRAGUE NORMAN AND
LAURA SMART NORMAN PROFESSOR OF PUBLIC HEALTH AND
PROFESSOR OF AFRICAN AMERICAN STUDIES, HARVARD UNIVERSITY

The depth and breadth of racial inequity in this country can be shocking even to those who consider themselves well-informed about social issues and committed to justice. Yet the data presented in this chapter by Dr. David Williams are clear—in most indicators, blacks, U.S.-born Latinos, and Native Americans do more poorly than whites. This is evident in housing, health care, the criminal justice system, employment, income, and wealth. Williams also documented an unbalanced scale when it comes to pre-kindergarten suspensions, pain relief, costs of bail, day-to-day discourtesy, and assumptions about honesty and intelligence.

It was that reality that prompted the vigorous discussion in the preceding chapter, *Fear and Despair: Consequences of Inequity*, about just how much concern should be dedicated to worsening mortality rates among a subset of the white population. But acknowledging longstanding patterns of racial discrimination should not mean pitting one marginalized group against another. Rather, they remind us that an interrelated set of social structures and systems has inequitable health consequences and need to be redesigned.

There surely can be no Culture of Health without fully reckoning with such disparities, and committing ourselves to addressing them.

Causes and Consequences of Racial Disparities

*Inequalities in health care are created by larger inequalities in society.
This is not random; it is the successful implementation of social policies.*
—David Williams

Health disparities by race generally fit within two distinct patterns. Groups with a long history of economic exploitation, social marginalization, and stigma in the United States—black, Native Americans, and Pacific Island peoples—tend to have poorer-than-average health. A different pattern is seen among more recent immigrants, notably Asians and Latinos, who initially tend to have better health, which worsens as they remain longer in the United States. The lower the socioeconomic status of these immigrants, the more rapidly their health declines.

Despite deeply troubling trends in much of the data about race, it is worth celebrating genuine progress where it can be found. In 1950, life expectancy was 60.8 years for blacks and 69.1 years for whites. Those numbers have moved steadily upward for both populations as a whole, reaching 74.7 years for blacks and 78.8 years for whites by 2010.

But a four-year life expectancy difference still represents a considerable gap. If life expectancy remained frozen for whites, while continuing to improve for blacks at the average rate of the U.S. population as a whole, it would take about 30 years before the age lines intersected. Another way to consider the magnitude of these differences: not until 1990 did blacks attain the life expectancy that whites had achieved in 1950.

Residential Segregation

We will not make progress in building a Culture of Health unless we begin to unpack and dismantle the conditions that segregation has created.
—David Williams

To understand the drivers of racial disparities in health, it is essential to recognize the influence of segregation over many decades. In 1944, Nobel Laureate economist Gunnar Myrdal called segregation "basic" to understanding racial inequality. The 1968 Kerner Commission agreed, terming it the "linchpin" of race relations. In 1982, John Cell, a Duke University historian, described segregation as "one of the most successful political ideologies" of the century, arguing that South Africa had copied the idea from the United States. Douglas Massey and Nancy Denton, authors of *American Apartheid*, called it the "missing link" in efforts to understand urban poverty.

Where someone lives determines the quality of his or her schools, housing and neighborhood conditions, their access to medical care and employment opportunities, and their ease of practicing healthy behaviors. Harvard University sociologists William Julius Wilson and Robert Sampson looked at 171 of the nation's largest cities and found that whites and blacks did not live in equal conditions in any of them. Their conclusion: "The worst urban context in which whites reside is considerably better than the average context of black communities." Whether the measure is access to social services, public transportation, navigable sidewalks, safe parks, or availability of nutritious foods, segregated communities tend to be unhealthy communities.

Segregation also drives inequalities in socioeconomic status. Black/white differences in income, unemployment, and rates of high school graduation could be erased, and racial differences in single motherhood cut by two-thirds, if it were eliminated, according to Harvard University economist David Cutler.

Income and Wealth

For every dollar that white Americans earn, Latinos earn 70 cents and blacks earn 59 cents, according to 2013 U.S. Census Bureau data. This income gap has long remained relatively unchanged—the same black/white differential was in place in 1978. Yet the gender gap in pay (women earn 79 cents for every dollar earned by men) has received far more public attention.

Moreover, income data significantly underestimate the economic divide, which is captured much more dramatically by wealth. For every dollar of wealth held by whites, Census data from 2011 show that Latinos hold seven cents and blacks hold six cents. Far from a gradual lessening of disparities, those figures have grown more skewed in recent years, reflecting the economic downturn and housing crisis earlier in the 21st century.

Socioeconomic status, as measured by income, education, or occupation, is well-established as a key driver of health. Indeed, research shows that it is a more powerful predictor than genetics, exposure to carcinogens, or even smoking. The lower the household income level, the higher the risk of premature death, with residents in the poorest households three times more likely to die before the age of 65, compared to the highest earners.

Similarly, education has a significant impact, both within and across racial groups. At age 25, whites with fewer than 12 years of education can expect to live 50 more years (compared to 47 for blacks) while white college graduates at age 25 are likely to live 56 years longer (compared to 52 for blacks). Incredibly, white high school graduates live longer than blacks with a college degree or more education.

As those data suggest, race intensifies the burden of low socioeconomic status. Why does race still matter so much?

Pervasive Discrimination

The subjective experience of discrimination is a source of toxic stress.
—David Williams

High-quality scientific studies conclusively document the persistence of discrimination in multiple domains of society. It is evident in the greater likelihood of being suspended from preschool, pulled over by the police, or arrested for drug-related crimes. Discriminatory practices also make it harder to obtain a bank loan, secure insurance, access high-quality medical care, purchase a car or home, hail a cab, find a job, earn a promotion, rent an apartment, and much more.

Beyond overt racism, a host of day-to-day indignities occur in the lives of non-white Americans. An Everyday Discrimination Scale measures some of those experiences, such as being treated with less courtesy or respect than other people; receiving poorer service in stores and restaurants; being viewed as dishonest, inferior, not smart, or a source of fear; and being subjected to threats, name-calling, and insults.

A powerful body of published research shows the health consequences of exposure to that kind of discrimination. A few examples, published by a single researcher, Tené Lewis, a scholar at the Rollins School of Public Health at Emory University:

• Increased risk of coronary artery calcification in middle-aged black women
• Among young pregnant women of color, a greater likelihood of having low-birthweight infants
• More rapid declines in cognitive functioning over time among older blacks
• Poor sleep outcomes among multiple populations
• Higher levels of visceral fat, which increases the risk of cardiovascular disease and diabetes

Other evidence shows that discrimination is associated with measures of inflammation, elevated blood pressure, and an increased risk of mortality.

Cultural Stereotypes

The racism that gives rise to everyday discrimination is deeply embedded in American culture. One place that is revealed is through the BEAGLE Project, a database of 10 million words (roughly equivalent to what an average college-level student reads over a lifetime), which allows word pairings to be examined.

Among the negative words most frequently associated with black: poor, violent, lazy, dangerous, and ignorant. A coefficient that captures the strength of these associations shows how closely they are tied together. This has profound implications for understanding what is occurring in American society. The police officer who perceives a black male as violent and dangerous is essentially doing nothing more than reflecting the norms that surround him, which have been deeply embedded in his subconscious.

A large body of research reveals that an individual who holds negative stereotypes of a given group will discriminate against members of that group. This is automatic behavior, taken without deliberate prejudicial intent, but the impact on racial and ethnic inequities is striking.

In a study of emergency room care at the University of California, Los Angeles Medical Center, researchers examined the use of pain medication in patients with a broken arm or leg. The findings: 55 percent of Latinos received no analgesia, compared to 26 percent of whites. Controlling for a host of other factors—whether the patient spoke English, severity of the fracture, arrival and waiting time in the emergency department—only made the ethnicity variable stronger. When the principal investigator moved to Emory University in Atlanta and repeated the same study with black and white patients, the conclusions were the same. And this pattern of minorities receiving poorer-quality care than whites has been documented across all areas of medical treatment.

And yet, as Williams emphasized, most physicians head to work every day seeking to do the best they can for all their patients. It is the deeply embedded racism of the culture that is shaping their behavior in ways they are likely not to realize.

What Can Be Done?

How can we address and dismantle this negative, racist culture that drives behavior in powerful ways?—David Williams

Ending his presentation on a powerful note of optimism, Williams reviewed some of the policies, programs, and practices that can generate meaningful change.

At the level of the individual, a seminal study by University of Wisconsin psychologist Patricia Devine showed that a well-designed intervention can help to break the habit of implicit racial bias among non-blacks. Key features of the approach she studied are education to raise awareness about bias against blacks and its link to discriminatory behavior, and training to apply bias-reduction strategies.

One of the learnable techniques embedded in the intervention is individuation, which encourages a focus on the distinctive characteristics of an individual, rather than on the social group to which that individual belongs. Replacing stereotypes, learning to take the perspective of a stigmatized group, and increasing opportunities for interracial contact are also part of that bias-reducing package.

The broader challenge of dismantling institutional racism requires, first, that it be viewed as a set of interrelated domains that together form an integrated system. A powerful paper by University of Washington sociologist Barbara Reskin argues that it is not possible to implement remedies for disparities without acknowledging and addressing that interdependence.

The subsystems of racism, in Reskin's analysis, include the labor market, wages, education, criminal justice, school segregation, residential segregation, credit markets, housing markets, and health care. Each affects, and is affected by, societal racism, but importantly, each also supports the others so that tackling any one subsystem only brings others into play, maintaining the status quo.

Reducing racial inequality requires forces that either act on every subsystem, or on key leverage points. Residential segregation is one such leverage point, where alleviation strategies ripple across multiple subsystems. Thus, Barbara Reskin concludes in the *Annual Review of Sociology*, "a systems perspective points to strategies to attack that system."

Importantly, strategies should be designed so that the disadvantaged improve most rapidly, narrowing gaps between populations. That priority, which is too often overlooked, can be understood by way of analogy to the tremendous progress that has been made in reducing tobacco use. While smoking rates have declined across the board, more educated individuals have quit at a higher rate, generating socioeconomic gaps between smokers and nonsmokers that are actually larger now than in 1970.

Numerous evidence-based models demonstrate that it is possible to reduce inequities when the political will to do so is in place. Examples follow in the areas of housing, economic well-being, and early childhood.

Place Matters

Among programs that have improved health by enhancing neighborhood and housing quality:

- The Moving to Opportunity Program randomized families with children to move from high-poverty to less-poor neighborhoods. A decade or more later, obesity levels and the risk for diabetes had been reduced in populations that moved.

- The Yonkers, New York Housing Intervention, designed to deconcentrate public housing, found that those who moved experienced better overall health, less substance abuse, less neighborhood violence, higher rates of employment, and greater satisfaction with public transportation, recreation facilities, and medical care.
- Purpose-built communities that employ integrative strategies, rather than a piecemeal approach, show a range of benefits. In the East Lake District in Atlanta, community leaders and philanthropists came together to address poverty, urban blight, failing schools, crime, and unemployment. Results since the 1995 launch of these efforts: a 95 percent reduction in crime; a 70 percent employment rate among able-bodied individuals, up from 13 percent; and 95 percent of students performing at grade level, up from 5 percent.

Economic Well-Being

Evidence shows that increasing income improves health, without any additional health intervention:

- The implementation of Social Security, and every subsequent increase in payments, has been associated with mortality declines for the elderly.
- The Great Smoky Mountain Study, which looked at the impact of a $5,000 annual cash supplement to Native American households following the opening of a casino, documented reductions in psychiatric symptoms among adolescents. The incidence of minor criminal offenses also dropped, high school graduation rates rose, and the racial disparities in both outcomes were eliminated.
- When the black/white gap in income narrows so do black/white differences in health. When civil rights and antipoverty programs took hold in the late 1960s and 1970s, blacks saw gains in life expectancy, declines in mortality that in some years exceeded those of whites, reduced rates of infant mortality, and fewer low-birthweight babies. But when the income gap widened, as it did in the mid-1980s, life expectancy declined in absolute terms.

Early Childhood

Investments in early childhood programs have powerful effects on health:

- In the HighScope Perry Preschool Program, black children, ages three and four, living in poverty and at risk of school failure, were randomly assigned to an intervention that included daily classes and weekly home visits. At age 40, those who had participated in the program were more likely to have graduated from high school and had higher rates of employment and home ownership, more income and savings, and fewer arrests.

- The Carolina Abecedarian Project randomized economically disadvantaged children from birth to age five to an early childhood program that offered a nurturing environment, good nutrition, and pediatric care. At age 21, participants had fewer symptoms of depression, less marijuana use, a more active lifestyle, and other educational and vocational assets. In their mid-30s, they had fewer risk factors for cardiovascular and metabolic diseases.

Reflections on Research

Ultimately, the health of America depends on the health of all Americans, and so it is in the collective interest to improve the lives of the most disadvantaged populations. Doing so requires greater knowledge of how to generate political will and inspire the commitment necessary to address the root causes of social inequality in health.

Williams' research revealed that Americans have rarely been particularly supportive of policies to help the poor, and are even less enthusiastic about policies that specifically target blacks. Scholars call this an empathy gap, and it has a long history. In *The Philadelphia Negro*, a study of black people published in 1899, W. E. B. Du Bois wrote: "The most difficult social problem in the matter of Negro health is the peculiar attitude of the nation towards the well-being of the race. There have, for instance, been few other cases in the history of civilized peoples where human suffering has been viewed with such peculiar indifference." More recent studies in the political science literature suggest a lack of empathy extends further, with findings that Americans have more empathy for animals and babies than they do for adults.

All of that speaks to the need to build a science base that takes seriously the challenge of telling the story of the disadvantaged in a way that allows Americans to connect to it. An early step is to raise awareness levels, since public opinion data show that most people do not even recognize the existence of racial inequities in health. As David Williams observes, "Many Americans think these are issues that are behind us because we've made such remarkable progress as a society. That is not where the data are."

Given the central role that emotion plays in policy preferences, the way in which racial disparities are framed and communicated has a powerful influence on the public response. The psychological literature reveals that words and phrases can be tweaked to tug more strongly on the emotional heartstrings, suggesting the importance of testing messaging to find out what resonates.

Around the country, there is evidence of interventions that make a difference, but less is known about how best to spread local success. Questions remain about how to scale up evidence-based programs for maximum impact; which strategies have the biggest ripple effects; and the sequence in which they should be implemented.

In discussions following Williams' presentation, one audience member emphasized the value of open dialogue in communities where research is conducted. "Thinking through patient-centered and community-centered outcomes is really key to building out into the community," she said. "These are really careful conversations to have." In particular, communities may be concerned about the use of control groups, and whether a study compares two effective interventions, or tests one intervention against standard care.

Reflections on Policy and Practice

> How can we get a Marshall Plan for disadvantaged communities in the
> United States so we can improve the opportunity structures in the places
> where people live?—David Williams

In general, the available research does more to document inequalities than to point to solutions. But enough is known about policies and practice that can guide action, and many of them save the system money as well. Ultimately, any approach needs to factor in social context because, as a World Health Organization report on the social determinants of health asks, "Why treat people and then send them back to the conditions that made them sick?"

During audience discussions, John Moon, MPP, who leads outreach and engagement at the Federal Reserve Bank of San Francisco, asked about community resistance to evidence-based strategies that were perceived as top-down. Again, the importance of building strong relationships with the community over time rose high on the priority list, with Williams emphasizing that communities are indeed willing to embrace scientific evidence as a tool to advance their cause. "I've never found rejection of scientific presentations," he said. "It depends on how you interact with communities."

Brian Smedley, PhD, executive director of the National Collaborative for Health Equity, who moderated the panel on which David Williams appeared, turned the discussion back to Moving to Opportunity. While high-quality evidence supports its value, he argued that other policy options are also needed so that residents can stay in communities where investments are being made, rather than face displacement as rents rise. "It's about housing choice," Smedley said.

Audience member Giridhar Mallya, MD, MSHP, senior policy officer at the Robert Wood Johnson Foundation, highlighted other potentially equity-building policies:

- The Earned Income Tax Credit, which provides subsidies primarily to low-income working families, has been shown to improve health throughout the life course, from birth outcomes to Social Security. The credit has rare bipartisan support, and expansion strategies are being considered at both the state and federal levels to offer larger credits and reach more childless adults.
- The Fair Housing Rule of the Department of Housing and Urban Development (HUD) requires communities to consider policies and practices that reduce segregation and promote mixed-income communities as they develop housing plans. However, it is uncertain whether adequate data are available to inform planning, and whether the rule will be adequately enforced.

With the end goal of building political will and influencing policy, audience members touched on a host of other topics. Among them: using legal mechanisms to drive change; capitalizing on the self-interest of private-sector payers; spreading research findings through social media; and bringing other lenses, such as the rural/urban divide, to the table as a way of leveraging interest in messages about health disparities.

Underscoring the theme of the session, Brian Smedley reminded the audience that inequity has proceeded "historically, deliberately, along the lines of race and ethnicity, to explicitly marginalize and weaken communities politically." While the process may be more implicit and less visible today than in the past, he said the need to "reverse engineer" the social engineering that has produced inequity is clear.

That will require the acts of many individuals, said Williams, quoting Robert F. Kennedy: "Each time a man or woman stands up for an ideal and acts to improve the lot of others, or strikes out against injustice, he or she sends forth a tiny ripple of hope, and those ripples build a current, which can sweep down the mightiest walls of oppression and resistance."

In a stirring conclusion, Williams spoke to his audience directly: "With the degree and extent of inequalities that are driven by mighty walls of oppression, we need ripples of hope. And it is my hope that each of you today would become a ripple of hope to sweep down the mighty walls of oppression and resistance."

How Americans Value Health

LARRY BYE, MA, SENIOR FELLOW, NORC AT THE UNIVERSITY
OF CHICAGO

DANTE CHINNI, DIRECTOR, AMERICAN COMMUNITIES PROJECT,
GEORGE WASHINGTON UNIVERSITY, AND JOURNALIST, *WALL STREET
JOURNAL* AND NBC NEWS

ALIA CRUM, PHD, ASSISTANT PROFESSOR, DEPARTMENT
OF PSYCHOLOGY, STANFORD UNIVERSITY

The challenges of confronting disparities, whether by race, educational level, or other measures, are highlighted by survey findings showing that Americans tend to see health as an individual, not a societal, pursuit. Although the vision for a Culture of Health puts well-being and health in the center of every aspect of American life, many people have yet to embrace this approach. Emerging research suggests that a broad commitment to community health and interconnection remains elusive.

The three contributors to this chapter—who offer preliminary survey results from a new nationwide survey on how Americans value health, a recent typology of 15 distinct community types, and research on the links between valuing health and healthy behavior—illustrate just how divided American adults are. This reality and these divisions, they explain, have important implications for creating policies, programs, and communication strategies that will move the Culture of Health forward and make health a shared value.

The American Health Values Survey

To begin to understand the health values and beliefs of American adults, Larry Bye presented preliminary results from a two-year, segmentation study funded by the Robert Wood Johnson Foundation.[1] Called the American Health Values Survey, this study by NORC collected data from 10,500 adults from June 2015 through February 2016. As Bye described it, "The goal of the study was to better understand how American adults differ in their health values and beliefs by constructing a typology of U.S. adults."

Collecting Data on Two Levels

Bye and his NORC team designed the study to segment or cluster adults based on their health values and beliefs by asking questions at two different levels:

- **The individual level.** Participants considered survey questions about: the importance of health as a core life concern; how they define health; self-efficacy when it comes to health in three domains (prevention, knowing when to seek care, and condition management); and trust in science and the health care system.
- **The societal level.** Participants were asked to consider questions about quality of opportunities to succeed in life and to be healthy; social solidarity; social and non-social determinants of health; health disparities; health as a priority for government and civil society; collective efficacy; and health-related civic engagement.

Bye said that this type of study—one that seeks to incorporate measures at both the individual and societal levels—had not been tried before. This two-level approach gave the study the best opportunity to establish a typology based on the breadth of ideas central to debates about health equity and population health.

Once constructed, the study was also designed to describe the resulting clusters against additional factors, such as: individual demographics; health status; tobacco use and body mass index; health care system utilization; insurance status; political participation; and political party identification and ideology. "The more we can understand how Americans differ, the more we can develop programs that are going to work and communicate effectively about them," Bye explained.

What Americans Believe: Preliminary Findings and Initial Reactions

A look at the sample-wide frequency distributions shows how Americans are divided over health issues and practices. While cautioning that the results would

---

[1] To read more about this grant, go to *www.rwjf.org/en/library/grants/2014/07/developing-and-implementing-a-rwjf-culture-of-health-baseline-se.html*.

not be fully prepared until late 2016, Bye presented these early findings and summarized his initial reactions.

Individual-Level Questions and Responses

- Do respondents make health a personal priority?
  - Always: 43 percent
  - Often, but have to put other things first: 50 percent
- How much effort do respondents put into preventing health problems by engaging in any of the following?
  - A healthy weight: 59 percent
  - Limiting stress: 54 percent
  - Limiting portion sizes: 51 percent
  - Exercising during leisure time: 43 percent
- Do Americans have an activist orientation when it comes to seeking care?
  - Able to speak up with a doctor, even when doctor does not ask: 67 percent
  - Able to get appropriate screenings or preventative care: 57 percent
- How confident are they when it comes to accessing care?
  - I know where to get care I need: 68 percent
  - I know when to get care vs. handling it on my own: 52 percent
  - I know how to manage conditions: 48 percent
  - I know how to prevent health problems in the first place: 41 percent

Bye's initial reactions were as follows: survey participants showed they were very confident about their ability to seek and find care, though they are slightly less confident when it comes to managing their health conditions and preventing them in the first place. Interestingly, two-thirds of respondents say they will engage with a doctor about a weight problem, even when a doctor doesn't ask about it. "Our typology is still a work in progress," Bye admitted, "but these are some of the important measures we're using. I'm not aware that anybody's tried to do this before at both levels, and we've been successful."

Societal-Level Questions and Responses

- Should the country make sure there's an equal opportunity to succeed and be healthy?
  - Yes, for equal opportunity to succeed: 48 percent
  - Yes, for equal opportunity to be healthy: 58 percent

- It is unjust if some have more opportunity to be healthy: 46 percent
- It is best for the country if people are concerned about needs of others, as much as they are about their own needs: 50 percent
- What non-social determinants of health strongly affect health? Americans responded "very strongly" to these:
  - Smoking: 76 percent
  - Stress: 65 percent
  - Personal practices other than smoking: 63 percent
  - Insurance: 61 percent
  - Health care access: 61 percent
  - Air and water quality: 56 percent
  - Genetic makeup: 40 percent
- What social determinants of health strongly affect health? Americans responded "very strongly" to these:
  - Jobs: 55 percent
  - Available food quality: 53 percent
  - Education: 45 percent
  - Community safety: 45 percent
  - The community you live in: 32 percent
  - Housing quality: 32 percent
- When it comes to health disparities in America, do you think individuals in the following three groups have it easier, about the same, or harder in terms of access to health care?
  - Blacks: 10 percent, easier; 45 percent, about the same; 30 percent, harder
  - Latinos: 14 percent, easier; 40 percent, about the same; 32 percent, harder
  - Low-income Americans: 13 percent, easier; 16 percent, about the same; 65 percent, harder
- What should be the Federal Government's top priorities?
  - Improve education: 52 percent, top priority; 40 percent, high priority
  - Reduce unemployment: 32 percent, top; 52 percent, high
  - Reform immigration: 34 percent, top; 37 percent, high
  - Reform taxes: 34 percent, top; 43 percent, high
  - Improve people's health: 32 percent, top; 51 percent, high
  - Address gap between rich and poor: 32 percent, top; 51 percent, high
  - Improve infrastructure: 27 percent, top; 53 percent, high
  - Address climate: 25 percent, top; 32 percent, high
- What should the government do to make Americans healthier?
  - Government should do more, even if it costs taxpayers more: 47 percent
  - Government cannot afford to do more: 37 percent
  - Don't know; refused to answer: 16 percent
- What are the priorities for your community and its environment?

- Make sure communities are healthy places to live: 21 percent, top priority; 56 percent, high priority
- Make sure affordable, healthy foods are available: 27 percent, top; 51 percent, high
- Provide safe, outdoor places to be active; 22 percent, top; 53 percent, high
- Provide decent housing for all in need: 25 percent, top; 50 percent, high
- Did Americans report health-related civic engagement in the last year?
  - Donate money to charity: 46 percent
  - Donate time to charity: 32 percent
  - Vote for or against a candidate based on a health care issue: 31 percent
  - Donate money or time to candidate/issue/organization: 20 percent
  - Contact elected official: 13 percent
  - Attend meeting: 11 percent
  - Contact media: 6 percent

Bye was impressed that respondents generally felt more intensely about most of the non-social determinants of health ("Everyone agrees that smoking is very bad for you," for instance) than about the social determinants, although all were viewed as strong influences on individual health. But that intensity dropped significantly when it came to the social determinants of health (such as jobs and healthy food availability).

> *You can believe that social determinants of health are very important, but yet not recognize that disparities exist with regard to race, ethnicity, and income.*—Larry Bye

Two findings gave Bye pause. Perspectives on the existence of health care disparities for blacks and Latinos in America "are particularly distressing data. Roughly 1 in 10 Americans actually thinks that these groups have an easier time." Bye noted there was a lot of work to do to overcome an "empathy gap," the same phrase David Williams used in the previous chapter, *From Disparity to Equity*, where he described attitude toward policies aimed at alleviating poverty, especially among people of color. Bye also pointed out that only half of the survey respondents said that the country would be better off if each of us were as concerned about the needs of others as our own. This "compassion measure" of only 50 percent, he said, is "a depressing statistic."

Lastly, Bye noted that there is a split between those who believe government should be involved in improving health equity and those who believe it is the job of the private sector or individuals. "There are strong differences of opinion about whose role it is. It is government versus civic society."

Early Observations on the Segmentation

Data analysis is currently underway, and final segmentation work for the American Health Values Survey was completed in late 2016. Preliminary findings demonstrate that:

- Six specific population groups emerged, each with varying views on personal health and the role of government. Bye named these six population segments to reflect their preferences: health egalitarians, equity advocates, committed activists, self-reliant individuals, disinterested skeptics, and private-sector champions. This typology of Americans' health values reveals that:[2]
  - *Health egalitarians* and *equity advocates* believe that personal health is of low importance and express strong support for the government to play an active role in health policy.
  - *Committed activists* believe strongly in the importance of personal health and support the government in playing an active role in health policy. For instance, 37 percent say they spend a great deal of time on exercising in leisure time (compared to 20 percent in the whole sample); 56 percent work on weight management (compared to 29 percent in the whole sample) while 53 percent work on stress reduction (compared to 24 percent in the whole sample). And 58 percent of committed activists (compared to 31 percent of the whole sample) believe that improving the health of citizens should be a top federal priority.
  - *Self-reliant individuals* and *private-sector champions* place a high importance on personal health and show less support for the government to play a role in health policy.
  - *Disinterested skeptics* give a low priority to personal health, and show little support for a government role in health policy.
- Bye's research on these six population health value segments further confirms that:
  - Some segments of the U.S. adult population are characterized by a high degree of health consciousness in their personal lives but this does not always translate into support of an active government role in health matters.
  - Some of these health-conscious segments possess a strong egalitarian ethos, and recognize the existence of disparities based on race/ethnicity and income, while others do not.

---

[2] For more information about the six specific population groups, go to *www.content.healthaffairs.org/content/35/11/1982*.

- Acceptance of the importance of the social determinants of health and the recognition of disparities is linked within some of the segments but not within others. In addition, some segments of those who are personally very health conscious tend to be highly civically engaged on health while others are not.[3]

When it comes to future research and practice, Bye noted that the American Health Values Survey should help identify the most important questions that change agents need to consider as they seek to begin community-level change efforts and make health a shared value. For instance, which segments are natural allies in this work and what might motivate them to provide support? Who are likely opponents? Are there opportunities to strengthen civic engagement among those who hold progressive public health views but who do not often participate?

But Bye admitted that some of the preliminary aspects of the survey might serve as cautionary red flags to those seeking to build a Culture of Health. Why? "We shouldn't make the mistake of thinking that people who are extremely health-conscious in their personal lives are civically engaged on health issues," he said. "Even more importantly, health consciousness in personal life does not seem to be very predictive of whether one has progressive public health views on disparities, other social determinants of health, and the role of government in health."

The American Communities Project

The U.S. is a big, complicated place, and we need ways to understand it, other than talking about what the U.S. average is all the time.—Dante Chinni

Dante Chinni admitted up front that he was different from other presenters at the conference, a self-described outlier in the world of academic analysis and health care research. This award-winning journalist with NBC News and *The Wall Street Journal* specializes in looking at data and demographics all over the country. Chinni's ability to "just kind of drop into some place in the middle of nowhere" and learn about the community, he explained, soon helped him realize that many places and demographics were remarkably similar, even if they were far apart geographically.

---

[3] Updated assessment from August 2016 statement on the American Health Values Survey: *www. nphic.confex.com/cdc/nphic16/webprogram/Paper37233.html.*

In other words, Chinni started to imagine his own typologies—not necessarily the rigorous, academic-driven typologies described by Bye in the earlier presentation but typologies that recognize that "this place is a lot like the place I went to before. It has similar kinds of people, demographic makeup, education, income, the economy is similar. And I began to think: Was there a way to take all of this kind of journalist knowledge and anecdotal knowledge and quantify it in some way?"

Forty Data Points, 15 Community Types

This is the way I see the world, the way I see the United States . . . like it or not.—Dante Chinni

Chinni answered his own question in 2013 when he helped create the American Communities Project (*www.americancommunities.org*), a combined political science and journalism effort that identifies new ways to look at and understand America's socioeconomic, political, and cultural fault lines that made the country what it is.[4] Under the project, Chinni divided the country into 15 types of communities and created "another way to explain who we are."

Working first with a doctoral student at Stanford University, Chinni identified 40 different data points or variables that would be used to create a new typology of the country. These 40 variables included everything from median household incomes and occupations to religious preferences, population, and race. "When we put them all together and ran them through the computer, we wound up with 13 different types of communities across the 3,100 counties in the United States," he said. With one addition to account for the largest cities, and another to split up a type that was particularly dense and large, Chinni ended up with 15 community types broken across the 40 original variables he used to cluster the different kinds of counties:

- *African-American South*: Home to 15.3 million people, these 371 counties running from Virginia through Texas are more than 40 percent African-American. The $35,561 median income is the poorest of the 15 types of communities.
- *Aging Farmlands*: Of the 576,000 people in the 161 counties clustered in the Dakotas south through the Great Plains, more than one-quarter are over

---

[4] Descriptions from *www.washingtonpost.com/blogs/govbeat/wp/2013/11/12/another-way-to-explain-who-we-are-the-15-types-of-communities-that-make-up-america/* and project website. Project statistical updates from Chinni's 2016 presentation.

62 years old and 96 percent are white. That makes the Aging Farmlands the oldest and least racially and ethnically diverse community type in the country.

- *Big Cities*: The 73.6 million people in the 46 largest counties in the country, which together hold the largest 50 cities, are some of the most diverse pockets of the population. More than a quarter are Hispanic, and nearly a fifth are black. The median household income is about $53,000, with large pockets of poverty as well as pockets of wealth.

- *College Towns*: More than one-third of the 17.9 million people in these 154 counties, clustered around college campuses outside big cities, have bachelor's degrees or higher. They are less diverse than the nation as a whole (85 percent white), and a higher percentage are between ages 18 and 21 compared to any other region.

- *Evangelical Hubs*: 12.5 million people live in 373 counties mostly scattered through the South, a high percentage of whom are religious adherents tied to evangelical churches like the Southern Baptist Convention. They are 85 percent white, and just 15 percent have a bachelor's degree.

- *Exurbs*: The not-quite-suburban, not-quite-rural bedroom communities in 222 counties are home to 32 million with a median household income of $63,000 a year. They generally lie on the fringe of major metro areas, in the space between suburban and rural America.

- *Graying America*: Scattered around the Mountain West and the northern border with Canada, extending as far east as upper Maine, more of the 15.3 million residents in these 364 counties are over 62 than are less than 18 years old. Median income is about $44,000 annually and the population is less diverse than that of the nation as a whole.

- *Hispanic Centers*: Based primarily in the Southwest, these 161 counties are places where self-identified Hispanics make up a large part of the population: 56 percent of the 11.5 million people identify as Hispanic, although they do not constitute a majority in every county. Most of the counties are heavily rural, but they also include large urban areas in Texas and Florida and up through Iowa. The population is much younger than the national average, with 30 percent under 18 years old.

- *Latter Day Saint (LDS) Enclaves*: The vast majority of the 3 million people living in 41 counties in and around Utah are white and young. More than three in 10 residents are under 18, and nine in 10 are white. LDS Enclaves are one of the country's least diverse types and the center of the nation's Mormon population.

- *Middle Suburbs*: About 16.3 million people live in 77 counties that ring big cities in the Northeast and Midwest. They tend to be less wealthy and less well-educated than people living in suburbs closer to the big cities (see *Urban Suburbs*, described below).

- *Military Posts*: The concentration of troops and bases means the 9.7 million people who live in these 89 counties are younger, more diverse, and more educated than in the average community type. Blacks represent 16 percent of the population, which is higher than average.

- *Native American Lands*: More than half the 695,000 people who live in 42 counties, mostly in the West, are indigenous Americans. They have the lowest percentage of whites, according to the Census Bureau, and their average household incomes are significantly lower than the national average.

- *Rural Middle America*: The 21.5 million people in these 599 counties live everywhere from Upstate New York to Minnesota's Iron Range. The small towns in which they live are heavily white and are not as reliant on agriculture as other rural counties.

- *Urban Suburbs*: The 66.2 million people in 106 counties just outside most major cities are starting to take on many big-city characteristics. Fifty-nine percent are white, 17 percent are Hispanic, and 14 percent are black. They are the wealthiest type of community, with an annual median household income of about $66,500.

- *Working-Class Country*: About 8.5 million people live in 337 counties that are among the most white (94 percent) and the poorest in the country. Many of these counties are rural outposts in Appalachia, though their footprint extends into the upper Midwest, the South, and parts of the Northwest states.

Chinni remarked, "All these places have different ways of seeing the world and different ways of seeing politics. They live in different environments."

Why This Matters: How People See the World in Terms of Health

The point is that community matters. We're living through a moment where there's just so much change going on . . . communities are moving in different directions. With the American Communities Project, I hope we have a way of understanding who we are as a country and, as time goes by, who we're going to be.—Dante Chinni

After reviewing these 15 community types, Chinni talked about "what this means in terms of how people live their lives and, in terms of health, how they see the world." Using 2014 annual tracking data supplied by Gallup, Chinni explained how the American Communities Project opens up a window into health-related habits that could be studied more closely in a Culture of Health context.

Consider:

- Do you use health insurance? The Middle Suburbs, Urban Suburbs, and Exurbs have the highest rates of insurance use, while Evangelical, African-American South, and Native American have much lower rates. The results were not surprising, Chinni said. "This is about how different the challenges are, community to community, what you're dealing with when you go from place to place."
- Do you smoke? While the national smoking rate hovers at around 20 percent, it rises to around 25 percent or more in Evangelical Hubs, African-American South, and Native American Lands, and drops in the Urban Suburbs below 17 percent. "When you're talking about need and what the different challenges are concerning health in these places—again, very different community to community."
- Do you have access to healthy food? (Or Who Shops at Whole Foods?) Chinni used shopping data about Whole Foods grocery stores from Experian-Simmons to drive home a point about self-segregation in population clusters. "People often say, 'Of course, people in Working-Class Country and Evangelical Hubs don't shop at Whole Foods grocery stores because there are no Whole Foods near them.' And my answer to that is, 'That's exactly right.' There are no Whole Foods near them and that's something to keep in mind."

Americans are self-segregating not only by political beliefs and attitudes but by where we shop and our health behaviors, said Chinni. "These things are indicators of what a community is like."

- What's your BMI? Based on body mass index (BMI), the project determined that 25 percent or slightly less of those living in Urban Suburbs and Big Cities are obese, while more than a third of those living in African-American South and Evangelical Hubs meet the threshold of obesity.

Reflecting a cornerstone of the Culture of Health—that health is a shared value—Chinni pointed out that obesity rates reflect more than what you eat. "It's about where you live. Are there gyms near you? What kinds of places do you have to shop in? Are there healthy food stores near you? But also, who do you talk to every day? What are your views about health? What are the accepted norms of the community you live in? These things are different, place to place."

Individual Beliefs, Healthy Mind-Sets

We found that simply valuing health is not a compelling motivator for behavior change . . . It's an empty value. It's not alive. It's not motivating, and it's not very compelling.—Alia Crum

For a conference audience looking to make connections between valuing health and actually changing healthy behavior patterns, Alia Crum's presentation brought sobering news: no such correlation exists.

Using research findings from her work as a psychology professor at Stanford University and director of health at Stanford SPARQ (Social-Psychological Answers to Real-World Questions), Crum reported that valuing health has no correlation with physical activity, healthy eating, smoking, alcohol use, sleep, number of medical conditions, BMI, or perceived health.

But Crum offered a solution to try and reclaim that connection: shift people's mind-sets about health. "I want to bring us back to the first Action Area of Robert Wood Johnson Foundation's Action Framework," she said, "and that is to create a shared value, and to change the beliefs, the mind-sets, the expectations that we have about health."

Mind-Sets About Health: Why Does It Matter?

Crum's research focuses on how changes in subjective mind-sets—the lenses through which we view and interpret the world—can alter objective reality through behavioral, psychological, and physiological mechanisms. Her work is, in part, inspired by research on the placebo effect, which demonstrates the ability of mind-set to elicit healing properties in the body. She is interested in understanding how mind-sets affect important outcomes outside the realm of medicine, in domains such as exercise, diet, and stress. More specifically, Crum aims to understand how mind-sets can be deliberately changed through intervention to affect physiological and psychological well-being.

Doing so, Crum said, could help address the fact that existing solutions are inadequate and that "Americans are in a pretty poor state of health . . . We all know there's a problem. One-half of adults have one chronic condition or more. That's one in two. We've spent so much money trying to combat it, yet what we've done is inadequate."

At the heart of Crum's research is trying to understand why these efforts have failed. Crum suspected that existing solutions to medical problems often don't work "because our actions fail to account for the social-psychological nature of the problem." Translated:

In order to motivate healthy behaviors we need to probe more deeply into the hearts and minds of Americans. The more useful question is not: Do people value health? But: Why do they value health? Why should we care about health, why should we value it, and what should get us up in the morning to actually change our lives to become healthier?

Attempts to Value Health Fall Flat

People are still defining health as an absence of illness.—Alia Crum

Using a multimethod research approach that included interviews and qualitative responses with individuals from across the country, Crum's study explored three questions: How much do we truly value health? Does valuing health predict health or lead to healthy behavior? What beliefs or mind-sets about health are most related to health and health behavior?

Here is what she discovered:

- Though an overwhelming 96 percent said they value health, only 64 percent put health in the top five in a hierarchy of values. "Over a third of the people have five other things that take priority before it comes to health, and only 16 percent place health as their number one value," Crum said.
- Valuing health does not predict health or lead to healthy behavior. The study found that valuing health has virtually no correlation with physical activity, healthy eating, smoking, alcohol use, sleep, the number of medical conditions a person reports, BMI, or perceived levels of health.
- If valuing health does not predict behavior, what does it even mean to say you value health? The most common response was "absence of disease" (37 percent) while diet and exercise was second (21 percent).

And though survey participants generally agreed that the overall health benefits include the ability to live longer and happier lives, Crum's study uncovered a fact that she said no one has really looked at before: namely, that the process of being healthy is "perceived as being unpleasant. That it's a duty. That it's isolating and it's depriving. And we found that this mind-set about the process of health actually predicts less healthy behaviors."

Changing Mind-Sets

With these new insights from the study, Crum determined that part of the problem causing health values to fall flat actually comes from focusing on the process.

If the process of staying healthy and valuing health is perceived as unpleasant and isolating, what would happen if one could change the mind-set to view staying healthy as social, indulgent, and even fun?

Consider two of Crum's examples:

- People who stand on their feet all day at work see this activity as burdensome, and it reduces the benefits. When they shift their mind-set to view working on their feet as good exercise, the mental and physical benefits (such as lowering blood pressure and encouraging weight loss) are more fully realized.
- When people perceive their foods to be indulgent (as opposed to sensible or healthy), their body responds more adaptively. Specifically, when people are told that the milkshake is indulgent, their ghrelin (the "hunger hormone") level is affected, which relates to more physiological satiety and faster metabolism than when they believe that same shake is a sensible, low-calorie shake.

Based on her research, Crum believes that we need to shift our mind-set about health from "static, end-state definitions that are seen as isolating, painful, and depriving" and move these mind-sets to a "dynamic process with health being an outcome of what we do and also a cause of the other things we value. It's inherently social, and it can be fun and even indulgent."

Reflections on Research

The challenges to understanding how Americans value health—through the American Health Values Survey, the American Communities Project, and the research on mind-sets—left session attendees with a myriad of questions.

Can We View Health Broadly?

To move toward a Culture of Health means deemphasizing individual or personal health in favor of public health focused on the collective good. But, says Crum, "people are individualistic and, at the end of the day, they're spending 24 hours with themselves." That's where changing mind-sets comes in—we can get "out of ourselves" by recognizing the benefits of health. An example is moving a mind-set focused on losing weight to a mind-set that focuses on how a person feels after exercising and how that influences others. "If we can change the feedback we're getting to focus not just on weight, you'll start to see the social benefits. And in so doing, we'll also be able to see that we are not just individuals in the end."

But Bye added that in spite of the cultural tendencies toward an individualistic viewpoint, there are sizeable segments of the population that want to support the Culture of Health vision.

Should Health Be Viewed as a Privilege?

One attendee, noting that she has health resources and the support of family and friends, spoke candidly about the "privilege" she feels when it comes to health because "I don't have to think about health because of the resources afforded to me." Chinni responded that thinking in terms of "privilege" is a very interesting way to conceptualize the ability to value health, pointing to data from Crum that shows how "white people don't think about community because they don't have to worry about it." After all, he noted, "the world is what you deal with every day, and that's not just true for health; it's about our understanding of other people."

Crum reminded the audience that half of Americans have a chronic disease. "I think we need to radically redefine health in an age when we're not going to be in perfect health all of the time. What does that look like?"

How Hard Is It to Change Mind-Sets?

Asked for an example of findings that showed a malleable response, Crum talked about changing mind-sets around stress. She pointed out that the American public is bombarded by messages about the dangers of stress. But when she created a three-minute video showing that the stress response is evolutionarily designed to boost our immunity and enhance performance, "those three minutes can help people change their mind-set. It's not all that hard to change people's mind-sets," she claimed.

Chinni was not convinced. "There are mind-sets that are locked in because of where people live, or by the kinds of people they associate with," he said. "Mind-set change can be done but a lot of work is involved. The key is it takes a long time."

This discussion panel, designed to look at research that tried to understand how Americans value health, closed by circling back to where it began, when moderator Len Nichols from George Mason University suggested that health care has become like food. As the panel started, Nichols recalled the act of gleaning described in Leviticus, wherein the landowner is admonished to leave something in the field after the crops are harvested in order to feed the widow, the orphan, and the stranger who happens by.

Leaving food in the field, Nichols said, is the same as making sure that all have access to health care: it's the ultimate community-building, stewardship activity. Crum called it the shared value question; Bye and Chinni referred to it as a necessary "dimension" in building a Culture of Health. And at the end of the panel, an attendee concluded that "this value of obligation to the collective good" needs to be more visible if the goal of achieving a Culture of Health is ever going to be realized.

PART THREE

PURSUING KNOWLEDGE
WITH PURPOSE

Research initiates the path to knowledge—knowledge that can drive purposeful action toward the greater good. Much on the research front today is in flux: technology, data, people, perspectives, and principles. Clearly, figuring out the best ways to manage, coordinate, and benefit from these transformations is a work in progress, as are the optimal ways to develop and use knowledge to build a Culture of Health.

The first three chapters of *Pursuing Knowledge with Purpose* consider the changing landscape of knowledge generation. *The Tyranny of Evidence* explains how relying on randomized controlled trials and credentialed experts, paying limited attention to systems, and other common elements of traditional research can actually frustrate efforts to establish useful knowledge. *Measure the Change You Wish to See in the World* explores models for understanding people's experience of well-being and how it is undermined by inequity. *The Secrecy Divide: Sharing Data Across Sectors* describes the "new normal," in which data sharing is viewed as essential to solving complicated health and social problems. The final chapter, *The Importance of Community-Based Participatory Research*, points to the growing recognition that engaging communities in the design and implementation of research that influences policy and practice is critical.

Navigating this evolving terrain requires a shift in traditional research culture. No longer will the researcher alone define the parameters and desired outcomes of investigations into the complex determinants of health and well-being. Community change agents and those who will reap the benefits—or suffer the consequences—of policy actions are increasingly recognized as integral partners in research development. Equally essential is collaboration among researchers from different disciplines, following different methodologies and research practices.

Expanding computing capability, new methodologies, and the advent of "big data" offer multiple ways to collect, process, interpret, and disseminate research results, and this new technological environment will require updated standards for rigor. Appropriate concerns about data quality, privacy, and ownership must not limit forward movement. And no one method will win out—different contexts call for different approaches.

Collaborating and sharing data with other researchers, communities, and individuals; making the best use of changing technology; exploring multilevel systems—all make for a truly fluid research environment, yet one that will be best positioned to contribute knowledge that can drive action across the Culture of Health Framework.

The Tyranny of Evidence

RAJIV MEHTA, MBA, MS, CEO, ATLAS OF CAREGIVING, AND
CO-ORGANIZER, QUANTIFIED SELF

BRIAN S. MITTMAN, PHD, SENIOR SCIENTIST, KAISER PERMANENTE
DEPARTMENT OF RESEARCH AND EVALUATION, AND SENIOR RESEARCHER,
VETERANS AFFAIRS QUALITY ENHANCEMENT RESEARCH INITIATIVE

KAREN PITTMAN, CO-FOUNDER, PRESIDENT, AND CEO, FORUM
FOR YOUTH INVESTMENT

LISBETH SCHORR, SENIOR FELLOW, CENTER FOR SOCIAL POLICY,
AND CO-FOUNDER, FRIENDS OF EVIDENCE

EMILY E. TANNER-SMITH, PHD, ASSOCIATE RESEARCH PROFESSOR,
PEABODY RESEARCH INSTITUTE AND DEPARTMENT OF HUMAN AND
ORGANIZATIONAL DEVELOPMENT, VANDERBILT UNIVERSITY, AND
CO-DIRECTOR, META-ANALYSIS CENTER AT THE PEABODY
RESEARCH INSTITUTE

Investing in the creation of evidence pays off. Evidence collected through sound methodological inquiry has contributed to significant improvements in well-being—medications that enhance our lives, cars that promote our safety, protocols that reduce workplace accidents, and more.

Yet, researchers, policymakers, and practitioners working to create a Culture of Health find themselves stifled and even tyrannized by some of these methods. Why? What happens when established scientific methods run into chaotic environments, confusing disciplinary and professional boundaries, and politically charged policy issues? What happens when researchers are confronted with complex interventions that contain multiple components, strong and highly variable contextual influences on outcomes, high levels of adaptation and instability in interventions and contexts, or other factors leading to extreme heterogeneity of treatment effects?

The five contributors to this chapter sought to understand how widely used methods for generating evidence can stymie and even block efforts to establish useful knowledge for a complex and changing world. Together, they highlight the risk of relying excessively on randomized controlled trials, failing to supplement those trials with process evaluations, or paying too little attention to populations and systems, and too much attention to the individual as the unit of analysis. They also warn against promoting one-size-fits-all interventions that lack tools to guide implementation, deference to credentialed experts over ordinary citizens, and an assumption of homogeneity across programs and people.

They also engaged with each other and with audience participants in further probing ways that conventional conceptions of evidence can limit understanding and ways it can be supplemented to promote insight and progress.

Evidence in the Context of a Culture of Health

When we're talking about this Culture of Health, we really are trying to improve things more than we're trying to prove things.—Karen Pittman

Attention to Nuance

Karen Pittman brought together evaluators from federal agencies involved with children and youth to "understand what these folks, who are charged with sitting at the intersections between policy, research, and practice, saw as the opportunities and what they saw as the challenges. The word that came up frequently is 'nuance.'"

Pittman is an optimist, noting that people care more about evidence now than they did in the past, but that this appreciation came about "with a hammer." That hammer is the randomized controlled trial.

Randomized controlled trials are often expensive, take a long time to yield findings, and may fail to accommodate the nuance required to understand social service initiatives. They do not work well when imposed on complex and at times only partially developed social interventions. Problems invariably ensure when policymakers feel they have no choice but to promote programs that have been evaluated in this cumbersome way.

The second problem is that communities might not be able to replicate an intervention that demonstrated its effectiveness through a randomized controlled trial. "When we send people to lists of gold-standard programs, which often had expensive implementation support, and tell them to operate that program on a fifth of the budget, they end up cutting essential things."

Off-the-shelf packages of programs that have performed well under tightly controlled protocols often do not answer practical questions, such as where, why, when, for whom, and at what cost does this work. "We don't explain what's essential and what's not essential. We give people the whole boxed set," said Pittman.

Why are answers to nuanced questions not available to communities that need them? Funders might not ask researchers to collect that information, or the information is not reported in the "what works" clearinghouses, or studies that find a program that worked for some but not all people does not pass someone's bar for effectiveness. "We have to be definitive and say 'This works well for this population in this circumstance, but don't do it over there.'"

A Bigger Picture and a Better Understanding

If we're going to get a Culture of Health, if we're going to achieve big out-comes, we have to focus on developing, experimenting with and spreading new tools, and maybe even harder, on encouraging a wider receptivity to a full range of useful and credible evidence.—Lisbeth Schorr

Lisbeth Schorr spoke about evidence needed to solve "wicked problems." This means being open to trading off some of the certainty that comes out of randomized controlled trials for a wider range of evidence that will produce more practical information to achieve bigger outcomes and solve broader problems.

Evidence of this type turns attention away from looking for isolated improvements in individuals to looking for a better understanding of population and societal problems. "Research illuminates place. For example, if research reveals that toxic landfills that ruin the health of children are more likely to be where poor people and people of color live, the underlying driver is not going to be a program—it is going to be a policy," said Schorr.

When researchers strive to support efforts to make an impact on communities or systems, they may find themselves in unfamiliar territory over which they have little or no control. Here, community organizations with limited infrastructures spend time and energy straining for scarce resources, addressing the multiple needs of residents, and juggling conflicting political opinions as to the right course of action. To succeed under these conditions, "We need evidence that comes out of ongoing disciplined inquiry among practitioners, policymakers, and researchers that is based on a deep understanding of the problem, of the system that produces the current outcomes, and of the detailed practical knowledge that is necessary to get good ideas actually to work."

Moving learning from innovative, small projects to achieve significant results among large and diverse populations—a move essential to creating a Culture of Health—requires new tools as well as new methods.

Citizen Science: Personal Research for Personal Benefit

Rajiv Mehta spoke to the value of "citizen science" in allowing people to choose the questions they want to answer for themselves and the meaning they assign to what they discover: "Citizen Science is the person himself or herself choosing the question to be asked, the methods to use, how to analyze the information, and the meaning they find from it. The end result is personal learning, which supports a Culture of Health at the level of each individual."

Citizen science uses scientific methods such as hypotheses, observation, experimentation, and evaluation, but it does not require "cyclotrons, white lab coats or PhDs." It is "personal research for personal benefit." The related Quantified Self movement (*www.quantifiedself.com*) is a loose community of people around the world who use mobile apps such as MyFitnessPal or portable monitoring devices such as Fitbits to self-track biological, physical, behavioral, or environmental factors in order to learn about themselves.

The underlying principle of both citizen science and the "quantified self" is that each person must have the capacity to learn and to improve himself or herself. This means that each must have access to personal data and the technical, social, and financial means to test alternatives and take meaning from them.

This level of personal control bumps into entrenched and paternalistic attitudes that stand in the way of people having access to their own data. It also challenges the systemic constraints that create obstacles in giving people the means to analyze and learn from what their data are telling them.

Citizen science aims to change this scenario. "When people want their data, we professionals should not get in the way. Moreover, when we discover or stumble upon tools that people could use for their own self-awareness, we should do what we can to bring those tools to the public."

Mehta offered a brief example from his research with Atlas of Caregiving (*www.atlasofcaregiving.com*), which is exploring ways to study family caregiving to make it easier and more effective. Using stick figures and simple lines, he mapped out care ecosystems, showing who was providing what kind of care for whom. Researchers and family members alike responded well to this simple "care map" tool, which was then described on a blog. Mehta is experimenting with teaching people how to create their own care maps and how to interpret them: "Just as the personal computer freed computing from the white-coated folks at IBM, a lot of new gadgets and technologies are allowing us to take charge of our own health in a similar way."

A caution about making data public and accessible: there is a danger that these technologies can be used for what some would call surveillance. "So basically our employers or our doctors want us to use the gadget so they can see if we're doing the right thing and then ping us. Such controlling approaches need to give way to a more democratic and empowered citizen science," said Mehta.

Methodologies for a Complex World

Asking 'does it work' or 'is it effective' is not a very useful question when we're dealing with complex interventions. The answer is almost always 'it depends.'—Brian Mittman

Meta-Analysis

Emily E. Tanner-Smith presented a case study of how new tools from meta-analysis can provide the kind of nuanced perspectives called for by Pittman and Schorr. She explained, "We can use new analytic methods to get at the key kernels or active ingredients of an intervention, and avoid the tyranny of homogeneity."

How can meta-analysis appraise conflicting evidence across primary studies? What can this analytic approach do to tease out key ingredients of programs and get at heterogeneity in a meaningful way?

Tanner-Smith analyzed findings from 185 studies of brief alcohol interventions for adolescents and young adults, using meta-analytic tools to identify which components of which interventions worked for which groups of young people.

Because they usually involve no more than one hour of contact time, the brief interventions are viewed as attractive, cost-effective strategies for addressing a public health problem. But they vary in terms of who delivers them, their underlying philosophies, their target population, and their therapeutic components or "active ingredients." Ingredients include goal-setting, strategies to moderate alcohol use, decisional balance exercises, and others. Different interventions use different combinations of ingredients, with actual components often tailored to the needs of the individual.

Using traditional meta-analytic techniques, Tanner-Smith found that across all 185 studies there were small clinical effects overall, but those effects persisted for up to one year. She probed further and in the next level of analysis used "meta-regression with robust variance estimation techniques, a recent advance that is useful in large reviews in which there is interest in prediction modeling."

Using this tool to examine each of the 185 studies for the presence or absence of each of 20 potential active ingredients and by going to the study authors for supplementary information, Tanner-Smith created a prediction model to answer, for example, "What is the predicted effect if we use a decisional balance exercise or not? If we use personalized normative feedback or not? If we use goal-setting exercises or not?"

She found that the decisional balance exercise and goal-setting were particularly effective for adolescents, an interesting finding since research suggests these types of cognitively oriented components may not be effective for adults.

The next step involved creating menus of "ideal programs," depicting, for example, how the most effective intervention might look for someone interested in working in a high school setting with adolescents between ages 12 and 15 who are already drinking at a high level. "Even though that intervention doesn't exist in the literature," Tanner-Smith explained, "we have used the information from these primary studies to create it. Obviously it is only observational, but that can be a very useful step for identifying types of interventions in specific settings for specific populations."

Tanner-Smith ended by noting that while her case study comes from the field of health, she is working with federal and state officials in criminal justice, education, and social welfare using the same approach.

Evidence and Complex Interventions

Brian S. Mittman offered responses to the question: How are complex interventions different from simple ones, and what are the implications of those differences for how we go about evaluating complex interventions?

"In simple evaluations, the key question is 'is it effective?' That is a yes/ no question," he explained. In other words, simple interventions and corresponding evaluation questions —"Is this drug effective?" "Should I include it in a formulary?"—are characterized by stability and homogeneity across settings. A stable context allows not only for testing effectiveness but also for understanding potential differences among subgroups of people or settings. When this is the situation, the gold-standard evaluation is the randomized controlled trial.

Complex interventions, however, have a number of characteristics that fail to meet the assumptions that underlie the randomized controlled trial, limiting the value of that method for generating complete, useful information. Complex interventions often aim to change human, organizational, or societal behaviors in dynamic, heterogeneous settings. Indeed, as organizations begin to implement these interventions, their learning curve may prompt changes in program context—the surrounding organizational structures and policies—and in program content.

"For complex interventions, the outcomes are often dominated more by contextual factors than by the main effect of the intervention. Often, we are not interested in the yes/no question. We are much more interested in what happens inside the 'black box,'" said Mittman. When this is the case, evaluators are challenged to provide detailed guidance in how to adapt and how to implement the intervention, and how to use insights into the "black box" of program operation and effects and impacts of the "black box" of organizational and environmental context. "If the answer lies not in the intervention but instead in managing the organization, perhaps the improvement we would like to achieve comes from careful attention to the setting."

The field of precision medicine offers a model for promoting recognition of the features of complex organizations and their heterogeneous effects because it holds that, unlike simple interventions, complex interventions have no robust, inherent property of effectiveness—there is not likely to be an effectiveness number attached to them. Other analytic tools such as structural equation modeling or path analysis can also be useful.

Mittman said that researchers tend toward randomized controlled trials even in situations where they are insufficient or ineffective because "we prefer methods we know how to use . . . we search where the light is, even though we didn't lose the keys under that particular light post."

Reflections on Evidence

The issues surrounding evidence illuminate areas ripe for further exploration and discussion. Some key questions are:

Is It Easier to Measure Progress in Some Sectors than in Others?

Probably yes. For example, "It is easier to measure grade-level reading than it is to measure critical thinking," says Lisbeth Schorr. Yet, funding streams influence the kind of evidence that is gathered, and narrow funding streams constrained by multiple conditions on their use can make it hard to gather evidence that gets to the when, how, and why questions.

Are Researchers Stifled by Skeuomorphs—Old
Techniques Applied to New Problems?

Eric Hekler, PhD, assistant professor at the School of Nutrition and Health Promotion at Arizona State University, introduced skeuomorphs as "taking concepts from an old technology and translating them to a new one." A note-taking app on a mobile telephone is a skeuomorph of a yellow legal pad, and a microphone icon is a skeuomorph of a three-dimensional microphone—both are images from one technology applied to another.

What are the skeuomorphs in current thinking? Building on a point originally made by colleague Stephen Schueller, PhD, an assistant professor of preventive medicine at Northwestern University, Hekler offered one example, social inter-ventions that require people to attend sessions in person, and noted that with smartphone apps, structured sessions are not necessary even though they have usually been considered essential components of programs.

Skeuomorphs are often useful because they help translate ideas from past contexts to current contexts, but they can also block development of new ways of thinking. What skeuomorphs—tools and methods from the past—might be frustrating new thinking and processes? The in-office doctor visit? Firewalled, peer-reviewed journals? Using programs as the unit of analysis rather than using practices within programs or systems surrounding programs? Randomized con-trolled trials?

How Do Federal Procurement Regulations Affect
the Ability of Researchers to Address Nuance and Use
More Creative and Effective Tools?

Laura C. Leviton, PhD, senior adviser for evaluation at the Robert Wood Johnson Foundation, wondered whether federal procurement rules are flexible enough to accommodate a level of nuance, given that proposals for funds are weighed through a system of structured numerical rankings.

People use numerical scores rather than judgment in making procurement decisions for a reason—numbers offer protection. "And the only reason to give up some of that protection is to get better results," says Schorr. A federal program officer has to have the backing of people higher in the agency to replace the pro-tection that numerical scores provide.

Dawn Alley, PhD, director of the Prevention and Population Health Group at the Center for Medicare and Medicaid Innovation, presented the funder's dilemma. If, for example, a study finds that an intervention appears to work in City A but not in City B, "I can't really imagine a world in which we say 'Yes, we will fund you here, but not there, because this works here and it doesn't work there.'" She hopes for a time when City A and City B each know what works for them because research has brought that information to the table.

There is some hope for a more flexible future. Pittman described an initiative in which several federal agencies streamlined their waiver review processes by allowing community organizations to submit a single waiver request. The consolidated waiver covers the services to be provided, the population to be served, eligibility requirements, and reporting. This simpler process frees up staff time and resources "so the community groups could actually pay attention to getting to the outcomes."

Schorr noted a new provision in the federal budget that acknowledges a role for judgment in figuring out what is working, when, where, and for whom. "So, there are little specks of light. I don't know how big the specks are, but there are some, and there is reason to be optimistic."

What Is "Good Enough" Evidence?

If complete evidence is not available, can researchers create "good enough" evidence for the person making the decision at a particular time? Is there a spectrum along which evidence can be created? "Without asking those questions first, people just apply a methodology randomly, and we just can't keep having conversations about the roulette approach to a methodology," said Pittman.

Shoshanna Sofaer, DrPH, MPH, director of Strategic Research Planning for Health Policy Research at the American Institutes for Research, is troubled by the tendency for researchers and funders to call for randomized controlled trials too early, before an intervention is fully developed. She suggests that "if something is too hard to implement, maybe what we need to do is find programs that are easier to implement."

Alley countered with a reality of policymaking: "When the problem and the political stream combine, it does not matter if the policy stream is not ready; the solution is going to get pulled from somewhere along that continuum. So I think academic researchers have to be prepared that sometimes what they have is going to end up being used as good enough."

When People Try to Take Charge of Their Own Health, What Happens to Traditional Thinking about Generalized Knowledge, Fixing Problems at the Systems Level, and the Limits of Self-Care?

Traditional science aims to explore what is true on average, but Citizen Science aims to learn what is true "for me." Is there a place for generalized knowledge within this frame?

Yes. Generalized data can provide guidance to individuals. Consider the model of national retail chain stores that operate under what look like cookie-cutter rules. These chains collect data all the time and pass directives to individual store managers. But, on the ground, the store managers use that data to do what they think is right for their store because they know that each store is unique.

The aims of Citizen Science and self-care are to learn and ultimately to act. But sometimes "you will find that you have run out of everything that's within your power to change," says Mehta. He elaborates, "So as much as I like to say I'm in charge of my own health, if I break a bone, I'm not fixing that myself."

Mehta described the root of his involvement with Citizen Science as "sheer orneriness." After hearing too many times that patients are noncompliant, he turned to the field of quality control for insights about fixing problems at the systems level. When faced with defects in an assembly line, quality control looks to systems, management, or the nature of the task. "Those are the sorts of things that technology is actually good for. And so I merrily started down that path. Little did I appreciate at the beginning how complex it was going to be."

When Stakes Are High and Findings Are Nuanced, What Guidance Can Researchers Offer Practitioners? Where Do the Clearinghouses of "What Works" Programs Fit?

Researchers in the field of meta-analysis are deploying new tools in order to tell practitioners, "You may not need to buy that $15,000 intervention package if we can identify the kernels that can be useful," says Tanner-Smith.

Mittman calls for algorithms that guide decision-makers in adapting programs to their settings:

> If I were given a choice of alternative packages of research evidence, one of which has high levels of internal validity, robust evidence of the form that clearinghouses require (such as evidence that this program has been effective in three particular settings based on well-designed randomized control trials), versus another program with extensive guidance in how to evaluate it internally and adapt it to my circumstance, but has less evidence or limited internal validity from research in other settings, I'd much rather have the latter.
>
> For complex interventions with heterogeneous effects, the likelihood that I will see results comparable to those seen in other settings may be quite low. I need tools to guide adaptation and implementation

of the program in my own unique setting in order to maximize the effects that I obtain for my own set of circumstances."

These thoughts call for reconsidering the many "what works" clearinghouses generated by government agencies and policy institutions. One participant views them as "stocking a pharmacy with drugs found to be effective, but then opening the door, letting people walk in, and telling them 'figure it out' without training the pharmacist."

Evidence can tyrannize, but it can also liberate. The generation of new analytic tools, the power of technology to inform knowledge in real time, and the excitement that builds when the interests of researchers, policymakers, and practitioners coalesce offer hope and promise for future knowledge building strategies.

|| 5 ||

Measure the Change You Wish to See in the World

SARAH BURD-SHARPS, MIA, CO-DIRECTOR, MEASURE OF AMERICA
OF THE SOCIAL SCIENCE RESEARCH COUNCIL

BRUCE Y. LEE, MD, MBA, ASSOCIATE PROFESSOR, INTERNATIONAL
HEALTH, JOHNS HOPKINS BLOOMBERG SCHOOL OF PUBLIC HEALTH, AND
EXECUTIVE DIRECTOR, GLOBAL OBESITY PREVENTION CENTER (GOPC)

KAREN MATSUOKA, PHD, CHIEF QUALITY OFFICER AND DIRECTOR,
DIVISION OF QUALITY AND HEALTH OUTCOMES, CENTER
FOR MEDICAID & CHIP SERVICES (CMS), CENTERS FOR
MEDICARE & MEDICAID SERVICES (CMCS)[1]

CARLEY RILEY, MD, MPP, MHS, FAAP, ASSISTANT PROFESSOR,
DEPARTMENT OF PEDIATRICS, DIVISION OF CRITICAL CARE MEDICINE,
CINCINNATI CHILDREN'S HOSPITAL MEDICAL CENTER, UNIVERSITY
OF CINCINNATI COLLEGE OF MEDICINE

Whatever the challenges of research design, the task of defining and measuring well-being remains central to erecting a solid foundation for a Culture of Health. In recent years, advances in approaches to measurement have improved our understanding of the critical importance of well-being in a society, community, or individual and how to track changes over time.

The four contributors to this chapter offer models for gathering data at multiple levels in order to understand how people experience well-being, how it is undermined by inequity, and how it can be nurtured through policy and practice.

---

[1] Material/content contained herein is representative solely of the author and is not to be misunderstood as an endorsement of the Department of Health and Human Services/Centers for Medicare & Medicaid Services.

Asking the Right Questions Through
Human-Centered Design

Policies and delivery reform models may not always be effective or responsive to the actual needs of the people they are intended to support. Why is this—and what can be done to improve the effectiveness of policymaking?

One reason is that we may not be asking the right questions or in the optimal ways, according to Karen Matsuoka. Human-centered design may help us do that. Originally trained as a health services researcher, Matsuoka spent the past year immersed in human-centered design as a visiting fellow at Stanford University's Institute for Design (the "d.school"),[2] where she applied the techniques of design-thinking to real-world health care problems in order to come up with patient-centered solutions.

Prior to attending Stanford, Matsuoka led several high-profile health care redesign initiatives for the state of Maryland. "Policymakers are being asked to think like designers without having a background in design," Matsuoka explained. "That's why I jumped at the opportunity to spend a year at the d.school, where design-thinking originated."

She found the experience "transformational." "In health services research, we are taught to adjust for 'patient non-compliance' and we use terms like 'hard-to-reach patients' and 'patient non-adherence'," says Matsuoka. "A human-centered approach flips that paradigm on its head. It digs deeper into that patient behavior to unearth what it can tell us about the solution we've designed and why it isn't working for patients."

What sets human-centered design apart from other design and quality improvement techniques is that it starts with—and continually comes back to—the use of robust empathy techniques to make sure that people's actual needs are being addressed in the design of policies and programs. In other words, "we need to ask what those needs are, and ask often." "When the solutions we've designed aren't yielding the expected results," Matsuoka continues, "more often than not, it's because we were asking the wrong questions and solving the wrong problem."

At the same time, patients may have difficulty articulating their unmet needs, especially if the solutions they seek do not yet exist. As Henry Ford once remarked, "If I'd asked my customers what they wanted, they'd have said 'a faster horse.'"

---

[2] More information about the Stanford d.school can be found at *www.dschool.stanford.edu/our-point-of-view/*.

As such, human-centered design approaches rely less on surveys and focus groups in the early stages of design and rely more on ethnographic techniques—such as in-depth interviewing, immersion, and direct observation—to develop testable hypotheses and low-cost prototypes about what patients want and need.[3] These approaches often call for co-designing with patients and providers to bring policymakers closer to the populations they are designing for.[4]

"Micro-experiments" can then be conducted to rapidly test these solutions on a small scale, using policy tools to scale and spread only those solutions that yield the desired outcomes and thereby minimize risk.

Identifying what works on a local level through rich community engagement is critical. Involving communities in designing and scaling their own programs will empower those communities to make real change and develop solutions that work.

Applying a Well-Being Framework to Measurement in the 100 Million Lives Initiative

The question that we're trying to answer is: whose life is getting better because we're here?—Carley Riley

Change agents in more than 100 communities in the United States and across the globe are collaborating in the 100 Million Healthier Lives (100MLives) initiative with a vision "to fundamentally transform the way the world thinks and acts to improve health, well-being and equity." The Institute for Healthcare Improvement (IHI) is leading the effort, which is committed to 100 million people living healthier lives by the year 2020.

Carley Riley is a member of the 100MLives Metrics Development Hub, which is tasked with creating a framework and measurement strategy.

The team has developed a conceptual framework composed of three interlocking pieces: health and well-being, equity, and sustainability. To achieve the 100MLives vision, health and well-being must be distributed equitably and sustainably over time. Population-level health and well-being requires the closing of equity gaps such as 25-year differences in life expectancy that sometimes separate people living only two miles apart.

---

[3] More information about human-centered design methods can be found at *www.dschool. stanford.edu/use-our-methods/*, *www.ideo.org/*, and *www.careinnovations.org/knowledge-center/ innovators-guidebook*.

[4] For more information, see *www.careinnovations.org*.

Measuring Health and Well-Being

The framework considers a healthier life as one that is longer and/or with higher well-being. Thus life expectancy and well-being are the two fundamental dimensions, with well-being composed of four domains: physical health, mental health, social well-being, and spiritual well-being. Moving from the conceptual to the measurable, the team developed a composite measure, WALY (well-being-adjusted life year), defined as one year of life lived in perfect well-being, based on the QALY (quality-adjusted life year) construct in health services research.

To measure well-being the 100MLives measurement team needed to design an instrument that was approachable, would be welcomed in communities around the world, and would enable the assessment of at least 200 million data points over time. The team developed the seven-item Common Measure for Adult Well-Being, which includes two questions to measure overall well-being, one physical health and one mental health question, two items to assess social well-being, and a seventh that addresses spiritual well-being. Key demographic data are also collected. After the *Sharing Knowledge* conference, the team developed an additional version of the Adult Well-Being Assessment.

The instrument has been piloted and its use in the 100MLives communities has begun. It is expected to change over time as the team learns from its widespread use. The team is also developing instruments to assess child and adolescent well-being. Coupled with the community-level measures discussed below, the 100MLives team members expect to learn a great deal about the determinants of well-being and associations among the many elements.

Measuring Equity and Sustainability

Equity includes two high-level measures: differences in well-being among groups and years of life gained. Multiple types of sustainability are measured, including financial, programmatic, environmental, political, resource, and leadership.

Measurement at the Local Level—and Beyond

Each of the 100MLives communities is creating its own local initiative with goals that matter in that community. Community-specific indicators might be related, for example, to healthy food access, high school graduation rate, or recidivism. In support the Metrics Development Hub team is crafting driver diagrams that map the community indicators into the larger 100MLives framework, which enables the community to understand how it connects to health and well-being on a larger scale.

Thus, to measure 100 million healthier lives many different drivers and many different outcomes on many different topics on many different scales and in many different places must be measured—a formidable endeavor! To manage this the initiative is creating a web-based platform, "Metrics That Matter Wizard," that communities can use to create measures, enter data, and view their progress. This will first be launched within the SCALE (Spreading Community Accelerators through Learning and Evaluation) communities[5] and then made widely available.

So, how do we count 100 million healthier lives? At the community and population levels by measuring changes in length of life and well-being and in WALYs, over time, and the equity gaps associated with these changes. And at the community level by counting the progress in the community-chosen indicators and creating a dashboard of metrics that communities can view and utilize.

Employing the Human Development Approach to Talk About Well-Being

Human development is defined as a process of enlarging people's freedoms and opportunities and improving their well-being.—Sarah Burd-Sharps

The Measure of America project at the Social Science Research Council provides tools for understanding well-being and opportunity in the United States. Project Director Sarah Burd-Sharps described the conceptual framework—the human development approach—used to talk about well-being.

The human development approach is rooted in the work of Harvard economist and Nobel laureate Amartya Sen. It was developed at the United Nations in the late 1980s and introduced in 1990. Central to the approach is a focus on people's capabilities—what they can do and what they can become.

The human development approach puts people at the center and considers everyday challenges in the interconnected way in which they are typically faced, rather than as separate problems requiring different solutions. It is an approach embedded in the concept of a Culture of Health.

In almost every country, with the United States as a notable exception, the human development approach is the gold standard for measuring well-being. More than 160 countries have issued reports that use the approach and the

---

[5] SCALE communities are 20 "pacesetter" and four "mentor" communities in 21 states already accelerating health improvement. SCALE is an RWJF-supported initiative managed by IHI.

UN-developed Human Development Index (HDI) to talk about well-being and disparities by race, ethnicity, gender, tribe, and so on.

The American Human Development Index

Measure of America has modified the UN-developed HDI to be more relevant to the American context. The American HDI comprises three dimensions, with associated measures:

- Long and healthy life: measured by life expectancy at birth
- Access to knowledge: measured by young people in school from ages 3 to 24 and adult educational attainment ages 25 and older
- Decent standard of living: measured by median personal earnings.

To create the HDI each measure is scaled and added together. The sum is divided by three and the result is a number from 0 to 10. The index can be calculated and compared by state, county, racial group, gender, etc.

The Well-Being Framework as a Support for Building a Culture of Health

Burd-Sharps offered a conceptual framework that consists of six ways in which approaches and measures of well-being can support and perhaps influence the building of a Culture of Health:

1. In this framework, health is considered a basic building block of well-being.
2. The HDI is very simple, but still has a lot to say. "You can really get an evidence-based conversation going about really difficult issues," Burd-Sharps remarked, such as how some groups in struggling areas are doing well, and vice versa. For example, whites in Mississippi (the state with the lowest HDI) have a higher HDI than blacks and Latinos in Connecticut (which has the highest HDI). What are the conditions, actions, and institutions that are creating such good conditions for whites in Mississippi?
3. A focus on well-being can promote fact-based dialogue on health equity. Work done by Measure of America in Marin County, the most affluent in California, found a life expectancy gap of 13 years between different parts of the county, and a gap of 11 years by race. The results led to a more objective and productive conversation about the reasons for these large disparities. As Burd-Sharps emphasizes, "These measures are critical for putting facts on the table and letting them speak for themselves."

4. A well-being framework can shine a light on public resource allocation. An examination of public systems—such as libraries in Sacramento or parks in Los Angeles—may show, for example, that in local areas of greatest need the facilities and resources are often meager. And those also tend to be the areas with poorer health outcomes, fewer youth activities, and other deficiencies in the elements of well-being.

5. Index rankings tend to stimulate a competitive spirit. The congressional districts with the highest and the lowest HDIs in the country are both in California: Silicon Valley (8.18 out of 10—long lives, high educational attainment, high incomes) and Kern and Tulare counties in the Central Valley (3.04—high levels of child hunger, extremely low crop worker wages). HDI advocates hope that Index results will encourage policymakers to invest in human progress through attention to well-being. We tend to pay a lot of attention to money metrics, such as stock market performance, GDP growth, and other financial metrics, which motivate investment in economic progress. We need to pay the same level of attention to metrics such as how long people are living.

6. Finally, the goal of index proponents is to translate the measures into action. In Sonoma County, Calif., that is just what happened. Working with the Sonoma County Department of Health Services, wine growers, crop workers, and others with a stake in county health, Measure of America produced a "portrait" report in 2014, in English and Spanish, that has led to a series of local initiatives to improve health, including passing an ordinance banning e-cigarettes in public places, mitigating tensions in some high-crime communities through public art projects such as mural painting, and a coalescing of the philanthropic community around using the HDI to decide where to focus funding.

In an illustrative example, after learning that the Census tracts with the highest and lowest HDI in the county in terms of well-being were just five miles apart in its largest city, Santa Rosa, residents launched "Hike the Portrait," an event in which people walked through both communities. Participants were so moved by that experience that they committed to the development of bike paths and other initiatives to bridge the two communities. This experience reinforced the validity of the work and the embedding of health in the larger community framework.

Using a Systems Approach to Promote a Healthier Culture for Children

Using childhood weight management as an example, Bruce Y. Lee described using a systems approach in promoting a healthier culture for children.

Major health-focused organizations have made recommendations around the global issue of childhood obesity. In the United States, the National Academy of Medicine stressed lifestyle factors related to diet and physical activity. With an international focus the World Health Organization Commission on Ending Childhood Obesity made similar recommendations, as well as others directed at market forces and factors, such as sleep, that interact with diet and physical activity.

Both entities emphasize taking a holistic approach in looking at factors that influence a child's likelihood of becoming obese, recognizing that obesity arises from complex systems—biological, behavioral, social, cultural, environmental, and others—and the relationships among those. "A system is a collection of components that are not independent. They're heavily interdependent and interrelated. Individuals do not exist in isolation. . . .. We have to think about systems when trying to develop solutions," said Lee.

The Dangers of Not Using a Systems Approach

If you don't understand the system and you're attempting changes, in some ways you're throwing things into the wind and seeing what might happen.—Bruce Lee

- Not addressing the underlying system can result in applying many unsustainable quick fixes to longer-term problems.
- Many secondary and tertiary effects may be missed. While missing negative effects can have obvious adverse consequences, missing positive outcomes may mean an overlooked opportunity to promote a policy or intervention.
- Well-intentioned policies may have unintended consequences when the policies are implemented in isolation from the larger context.
- Time, effort, and financial and other resources may be expended needlessly as a result of nonproductive trial and error.

The Challenges of Taking a Systems Approach to Change

- Other factors and mechanisms may not have been considered. National Academy and WHO recommendations have focused on diet and physical activity in addressing childhood obesity. Yet, other studies have indicated a possible link between medication use and subsequent obesity development.
- Taking into account the time lag of effects can be daunting. For example, dealing with the effects of maternal factors on early childhood means looking at the mothers' development, environment, and the factors affecting them before, during, and for some time after birth. In studying what happens after

birth many factors and relationships may be missed if what happens before birth is not considered.

- How different policies and interventions fit together has implications for outcomes. Often they are considered individually, but their collective operation may be helpful, synergistic, or negative.
- Without an understanding of existing heterogeneity it can be difficult to know where to apply different policies and interventions. While people are connected in many ways, they also have numerous differences —racially, ethnically, socioeconomically, culturally, and so on. These differences can have important implications for policy and practice.

It can be difficult to know how to implement different policies and what the potential impact will be. A systems approach can help.

Lee described a geospatially explicit simulation model for obesity, similar to the computer game SimCity, in which an entire community is mapped for food sources (grocery stores, corner stores, restaurants) and physical activity locations (parks, recreation centers, gyms). Adults and children of all ages are also mapped and placed in households. Model users can track people as they travel through their day, from home to school or workplace, passing by food stores and physical activity locations and making decisions as they go about eating, exercise, etc. Each virtual person is embedded with a metabolic model so that their eating and activity decisions—calories in and calories out—can be translated into change in body mass index.

The model can be used to test different policies and interventions and the relationships and outcomes between them. Results can inform policy and intervention design and implementation. Real-life experience will generate more results to update the model.

This model was used to advise decision-making on an urban farm bill before the Baltimore City Council. Testimony at a public hearing showed expected outcomes if the bill were implemented, based on simulation runs of the model. The bill passed in part because evidence from the model provided support.

A systems approach has transformed many other fields, such as meteorology, transportation, and air traffic control. The model described is just one example of how a systems approach can help transform how not just childhood obesity is addressed but child health and, indeed, overall health.

Reflections on Research

Efforts are underway globally to assess well-being at individual, community, and societal levels, and to compare levels of well-being by dimensions that include geography, race, ethnicity, gender, socioeconomic status, and so on. The validity of these efforts will be bolstered by further work in several areas:

- **Filling gaps in measurement:** What is missing from the conversation that should be captured?
- **Self-reported measurement:** Carley Riley stressed the importance of "valuing the self-reported measure as one of great meaning." But the gap between recognizing the value of the self-reported measure and implementing it on a large scale is hard to fill, although critical to understanding well-being.
- **Measurement of social health and the social part of well-being:** Communities are looking for ways to understand how community members experience social connectedness, belonging, community pride, and, conversely, social isolation. Riley has seen a need for a robust measurement framework in this area.
- **Development of mental health indicators:** Sarah Burd-Sharps noted the dearth of data on all aspects of mental health.
- **Measurement of civic engagement:** Little information is available on how residents are involved with their communities, beyond voting statistics. This area also warrants more attention to measurement, according to Burd-Sharps.
- **Understanding the appropriate role of spending measures:** Are measures of health care spending useful measures of access or do they get in the way of measuring actual results? Spending can be an important metric not as an outcome but as a contribution to the conversation about value for resources—what results we are getting in relation to how resources are allocated. This may influence how resources can be utilized in the future to support healthier lives.
- **Probing the role of race and ethnicity:** How are patterns of segregation, desegregation, and resegregation changing? What is the impact of these changing patterns on well-being by race and ethnicity—and also by gender and race criteria (e.g., comparing black women), where significant disparities are often unaddressed? It is important to understand these changing dynamics and how society and communities can respond and shape the related outcomes.
- **Enhancement of the Behavioral Risk Factors Surveillance System (BRFSS):** The BRFSS provides a wealth of information about health-related risk behaviors, chronic health conditions, and use of preventive services among adults in the United States. Further enhancement of the system would offer the potential for a life course perspective (e.g., effects of life challenges or economic disadvantages over time). The 100MLives Metrics Hub team is considering ways to leverage the platform and develop it as an even richer resource for understanding communities and individual lives.

- **Integrating more social and emotional factors into studies of childhood obesity and other health issues**: How can such factors be incorporated into thinking on these issues? A sensitivity analysis can show if they might be game-changers on whether an intervention works or not, according to Bruce Lee, even if the intervention is not based on behavioral or social factors.
- **Aligning measures of well-being:** What can be done to bring consistency to the various models and measures of well-being? Different models may be addressing different elements of the issue—for example, measuring well-being as an outcome versus measuring the context that may create well-being. That said, there is desire for measurement commonality and enthusiasm for a strong well-being index.
- **Developing more linkages among data sets, models, and output**: This will require addressing the technological and operational gaps that prevent such connections as well as cultural gaps related to different disciplines working within the same areas. Common technology and common language are needed, as is further discussed in the next chapter, *The Secrecy Divide: Sharing Data Across Sectors*.
- **Accounting for uncertainty in models of well-being:** How can uncertainty be addressed in models with substantial uncertainty, both from sampling and from unmeasured confounders? The model-building process can be as important as running the model, Lee emphasized. Decision-makers, policymakers, and others must join designers in model-building that requires understanding the factors involved, the different relationships, and what is known and not known. An iterative process of testing different parameters can help the group understand the system and move toward solutions.
- **Handling the complexity of complicated systems models:** As multiple factors are introduced, what is the effect on the model's predictive ability and validation? Here too the process is key. By progressively building the model, adding complexity in layers, each level and each iteration can be validated, even as the model becomes more complex. This involves fine-tuning, removing a factor, seeing what happens, and then seeing what happens when it is added back. It is both a science and an art.

Reflections on Policy and Practice

The value of models, approaches, indices, and systems for measuring well-being is in their use to guide policymaking and program development. How can designers of these measures ensure that their efforts will make a substantial contribution to improving people's health and well-being?

The answer is rooted in threading the process of measure design through measure implementation and interpretation to responsive action with the technical expertise and knowledge of researchers, broad political overview of policymakers, and on-the-ground experience, know-how, and enthusiasm of local change agents and community members. As Sarah Burd-Sharps observed, "There is a hunger for data. There's a hunger for dashboards that help elected officials monitor how they're doing on the things that they've committed to."

The interest is there among policymakers, officials, and community leaders. The key is to choose partners carefully and build a process where multiple stakeholders work together. The most carefully crafted model will only have meaning and be used to help change policy, programs, and the way things are invested if people embedded in a community are willing and able to see the process through. "Where that happens," said Burd-Sharps, "we're able to watch incredible progress." Without it, there is not the capacity or political will to accomplish what needs to be done.

To do this requires involving people in measurement design, so models developed reflect real-life experience, needs, and demands. And it means building "local capacity to understand, select, and use metrics that matter to drive local change," Carley Riley stressed. These are metrics that drive quality improvement at a fast pace but also offer the ability to track community effects over time. "That process is one not only of figuring out how to get the data at the right level in the right time scale, and the right way that resonates and matters and drives change, but then also how do we build that local understanding and capacity to actually use that data in a way that creates healthier lives," said Riley.

So, for example, while the HDI is a summary, reductionist measure in order to allow comparisons across communities and groups, the process of preparing community reports using the HDI is "deeply participatory and inclusive," said Burd-Sharps. Pains are taken to ensure that the voices of marginalized and often excluded people and organizations are reflected. A highly diverse advisory committee contains both "the usual suspects" as well as those often not at the table.

Broadening the type of data collected—to include not only quantitative but also storytelling and other qualitative data, as well as visual imagery such as photos, drawings, and rich pictures—will increase the likelihood of identifying the data that matter and actually shape the narrative and inspire action.

Including those who can make change and are affected by change in the design of measures and models of well-being and ensuring that they have the will and capacity to put these measures to use will not only appropriately measure well-being but help bring greater well-being to more people over time.

6

The Secrecy Divide

Sharing Data Across Sectors

HEATHER JOSEPH, MA, EXECUTIVE DIRECTOR, SPARC (SCHOLARLY
PUBLISHING AND ACADEMIC RESOURCES COALITION)

JOSHUA M. SHARFSTEIN, MD, ASSOCIATE DEAN FOR PUBLIC HEALTH
PRACTICE AND TRAINING, JOHNS HOPKINS BLOOMBERG SCHOOL
OF PUBLIC HEALTH, AND FORMER SECRETARY, MARYLAND DEPARTMENT
OF HEALTH AND MENTAL HYGIENE

STEVEN H. WOOLF, MD, MPH, DIRECTOR, CENTER ON SOCIETY AND
HEALTH, AND PROFESSOR, DEPARTMENT OF FAMILY MEDICINE AND
POPULATION HEALTH, VIRGINIA COMMONWEALTH UNIVERSITY

As measurements of well being become more sophisticated, the value of thoughtful information sharing to inform cross-sector solutions escalates. From the federal government to state and local governments, from academia to community action groups, from the public health department to the police department, a new normal is evolving in which sharing health data among sectors is viewed as not only acceptable but essential to solving complex health and social problems and advancing toward a true Culture of Health that encompasses all.

But progress toward the new normal faces serious challenges. The three contributors to this chapter address some of the apprehensions that the changing information environment brings, while being clear that the secrecy divide has been bridged and a new age of data sharing is here to stay.

Bringing a Sea Change to Federal Data-Sharing Policy

On his first full day in office, January 21, 2009, President Barack Obama issued a Presidential Memorandum on Transparency and Open Government, which instructed the director of the Office of Management and Budget, the chief technology officer, and the administrator of the General Services Administration to develop an Open Government Directive within 120 days.

The Directive set the tone for a landmark shift in how data are handled, according to Heather Joseph, and established new expectations for transparency and openness in government activities and outputs, including information and data.

The Administration took further action to bolster federal policy requiring the sharing of data with two instructions issued in 2013. A February memorandum from the director of the White House Office of Science and Technology Policy required that all federal agencies with more than $100 million in the conduct and funding of scientific research create policies for the open sharing of research products, including data. And in May the president issued an Executive Order—Making Open and Machine Readable the New Default for Government Information.[1]

As federal agencies have moved into a new era of openness, so have other public and private funders, including large foundations. Now, a plan for sharing the outputs of research more freely is a routine requirement of funding proposals, resulting in a recalibration of the way that researchers think about the collection and use of data. As Joseph observes, "We're starting to live in a world where we can think about the norm moving from holding our data close unless there's a compelling reason to share it, to 'our data is open unless or until we can articulate a compelling reason to keep it locked up.'"

Events like the Ebola pandemic, the Zika crisis, and the National Cancer Moonshot led by Vice President Biden elicit calls for the wide sharing of relevant data in order to bring all resources to bear on serious and complex problems. Thus, data-sharing policies and requirements, far from being punitive, are propelled by the belief that opening up data to broad use "will accelerate leaps of science; fuel discovery; speed up the translation of results into services, into treatments, into cures; fuel the economy—all things that feed the public good," said Joseph.

Yet, the open sharing of data can be hindered by challenges in meshing incongruent and often proprietary technologies, by regulatory and organizational limitations, and by commercialization concerns. "We often find ourselves just staring inertia and slow-changing cultural norms and practices back in the eye," said Joseph.

---

[1] For more on federal health data sharing initiatives visit *www.healthdata.gov*. Also see *www. healthdatapalooza.org* for information on Health Datapalooza, a national conference on the sharing and use of health data.

Sharing Data in Academia and Public Health: Examples and Principles

Contributing Academic Knowledge to Support a City's Future

After the death of Freddie Gray on April 19, 2015, as a result of injuries incurred during transport by police, the city of Baltimore experienced significant protests and ongoing unrest. Spurred by these events staff at the Johns Hopkins Bloomberg School of Public Health began thinking about what the school could do to provide better support to the city. Courses at the school talk about Baltimore. Students write papers about Baltimore. Surveys are done. But these were not generally made available to the Baltimore community (an issue explored more fully in the next chapter, *The Importance of Community-Based Participatory Research*).

To remedy this situation, each department and the Office of the Dean has developed a mission statement for its relationship with the city as well as a project to further that mission. In one project researchers are helping the Police Department use data more effectively to reduce violence and to improve relations with the community. "Universities should be thinking about data sharing . . .," Joshua Sharfstein posits, "and not just the data sets that they're doing, but all the knowledge that they're generating, the analysis."

In another outreach initiative researchers are participating in Open Baltimore (*www.data.baltimorecity.gov*), the city's effort to make data sets from many sectors (health, public safety, housing, finance, culture and arts, transportation, and others) available to the community. "There's a huge amount of enthusiasm for that from the community organizations we deal with," said Sharfstein. "You would be surprised what people can pull off when they have access to things."

Broadening the Reach of Public Health with Cross-Sector Data

With research or clinical use of data there is an expectation of consent when the data are identifiable to an individual. That is not so much the case with public health data. Public health considers data use as a public good. Certain things are reportable to the health department and individuals do not have the option to consent or not, Sharfstein noted. Sharfstein previously served as secretary, Maryland Department of Health and Mental Hygiene, and earlier as commissioner of health, Baltimore City.

The right of a health department to collect certain identifiable data brings clear responsibilities: the department must keep such data private and use them well. To do otherwise would delegitimize the health department's work. Sharfstein elaborates, "From a health department's perspective, it's identifiable data that you want. You don't just want to know Census tract. You want to know block. You don't just want to know that individuals over 65 have a greater risk of whatever. You want to be able to help them. You want to know who it is."

An example of the public health use of data is an effort to include school absenteeism data from the Baltimore school district in the Maryland Health Information Exchange.[2] Many studies have connected absenteeism to a variety of health outcomes for children, according to Sharfstein. With such data available pediatricians and nurse practitioners could consider absenteeism as a vital sign. But since this information is identifiable (and needs to be identifiable for the provider working at the patient level) there are regulations that inhibit the flow of the information.

Another example is the use of Health Information Exchange data on falls by older adults as part of a city-wide campaign—Baltimore Falls Reduction Initiative Engaging Neighborhoods and Data (B'FRIEND)[3]—to reduce falls by one-third over three years. With a clear public health goal the city health department will be able to obtain the data, but rules will still apply to its use and legal agreements will be required.

Sharfstein delineated principles for public health sharing of identifiable data when addressing "a really difficult health problem":

- There must be a clear public health goal, with a plan to use the data to improve health.
- Use of identifiable health information must be limited to what is needed and only shared with the minimal number of people necessary to meet the goal.
- Legal agreements that require the data to be used only for the intended purpose must govern data use.
- There must be a clear benefit to the individuals attached to the data (e.g., helping a child stay in school or assisting those who experience falls).
- Data use, and its impact on public health, should be transparent. People have a right to know how the data are being used and whether that use is working.
- Public input must be part of developing proposals for data sharing.

---

[2] The Maryland Health Information Exchange links all of the state's acute care hospitals as well as approved physicians' offices and other health organizations in a statewide system that allows instant and secure sharing of health information. Maryland is the first state to attain this level of connectivity.

[3] B'FRIEND is supported by a grant from the Robert Wood Johnson Foundation through its program Data Across Sectors for Health (DASH).

Meeting these principles will foster understanding about why and how data will be used and the outcomes that the data sharing is designed to produce. "If it can truly be for action, if somebody's going to be using that data in a certain way and can speak to that and has credibility," said Sharfstein, "that's the locomotive that pulls things forward."

Applying Big Data and Advanced Computing Techniques to Improve Population Health

Two emerging and connected trends—"big data" and supercomputing—allow for deep dives into data and open the door to blending data across fields. Steven Woolf described how each, separately and together, offers potential for strengthened and more thorough and responsive research and policy.

Big data (very large data sets that require sophisticated software tools to collect, manage, process, and analyze) that are useful in the health arena may include environmental, genomic, microbiome, medical record, personal health, public health, and other data sets. With new analytic methods these data can be mined for fresh and integrated insights previously not available. Instead of working with a priori hypotheses, data are analyzed by computer and then exploratory questions are identified.

The availability of big data and the tools and methods to take full advantage of it leads to the potential for layering many kinds of data to allow for comprehensive studies of the return on investment for a range of interventions. For example, an investment in improving education can also lead to improvements in health, better jobs, lower crime rates, economic development, increased tax revenues, and lower demand for social services. To demonstrate the collective impact of such an investment requires combining data from a wide range of sources: education, health care, employment, law enforcement, tax systems, social services, and so on.

Also needed to make this work in real-world situations are a common agenda, shared measurement plans and tools, mutually reinforcing activities, and ongoing communication among the various parties involved. Woolf offered the Build Healthy Places Network (*www.buildhealthyplaces.org*) as an example of a collaborative effort to do that. The Network connects leaders and practitioners, curates resources, and builds the knowledge base to support cross-sector collaboration to improve low-income communities and the lives of people living in them.

Woolf identified five domains that shape health outcomes: health systems, health behaviors, socioeconomic factors, physical and social environments, and public policies and social spending (Box 6.1). Each offers an opportunity for a

Box 6.1

Live Well San Diego (*www.livewellsd.org*) is a collaboration of county government, businesses, community- and faith-based organizations, schools, health care and technology providers, law enforcement and the courts, active military and veterans, and others united in a vision to improve the health, safety, and well-being of all residents of San Diego County. The initiative has taken a data-driven approach to accomplishing its goals.

Woolf leads a demonstration project to examine how big data can support public health and social policy within a defined geographic area, with San Diego as the test case. The project includes establishing a "big data repository" that will support the integration of data from multiple sectors in San Diego, while ensuring the security of the data and addressing the challenges of interface across disparate data architectures. The goal is to explore whether community decisions can benefit from technologically advanced methods for displaying, analyzing, and modeling local data from health care, public health, social services, the environment, and other domains.

deep dive into existing data sets: "We can use data to find out what happened, analyze why it happened and develop models of what will happen—and optimization to get the best bang for the buck."

Reflections on Data Sharing

Consideration of data sharing among researchers, across sectors, and across geographies raised a set of issues and questions among session attendees.

Encouraging Researchers to Share Data—Clean and Useable Data—Promptly

Often researchers are reluctant to share data before they have published everything they can from the data. How can researchers be incentivized to share data much earlier, before they have exhausted all publication possibilities?

At Bloomberg School of Public Health Sharfstein has promoted a philosophy that it's not enough to simply support the idea of data sharing but that the school has a responsibility to the city of Baltimore "to make data available because people in the city can use it."

Publications are a key component of an individual's curriculum vitae when being considered for academic promotion and tenure. Including the sharing of data sets, and the use of one's data by others, as criteria for promotion would likely provide an incentive to do just that. Heather Joseph said that SPARC is working on a campaign called Change the Form, which asks universities to include in their tenure guidelines questions such as: "Have you made your data sets open? How have you shared your data?"

Data curation is also critical—ensuring that the data shared are, in fact, clean, annotated, and actually useable. Joseph expressed concern about how to get researchers to do that work, noting that the better the data, the better the output of the university, the better the university looks, and the fuller the contribution to better outcomes wherever the data are shared. She concluded, "You need to have people rewarded and recognized . . . It's a big culture change."

Sharing Health Data with Other Sectors

Health researchers and professionals seek to share data from other fields, such as education or law enforcement. What about the sharing of health data with other sectors?

Several issues may be at play here. Asking, for example, a school district to share absenteeism data with health care providers while those providers refuse to share student health data with the school system could be viewed as a "massive hypocrisy," Joshua Sharfstein acknowledged. In such a case, a clear understanding of the purpose for the data sharing would be essential, as would legal agreements to govern the sharing arrangement. But there is not necessarily "perfect reciprocity," he noted.

An important role for public health in the future, Sharfstein predicted, is likely to include addressing goals that, while perhaps not directly health-focused, are nevertheless important factors in building and maintaining a local Culture of Health, such as decreasing community violence, keeping youth in school, and improving housing conditions. Public health systems have the skills to meld data from other sectors to further such goals. But, he said, "Certainly the value of that sharing should go back to the other agencies one way or another."

Sharfstein cited an example from his tenure as Baltimore Health Commissioner. While reviewing medical examiner data on drug overdoses for a project to develop strategies to reduce heroin overdose deaths in Baltimore, researchers noticed a huge spike in cocaine deaths during the previous year. Police were asked, "Any idea why we had this huge spike?" They replied, "Last year? Cocaine was everywhere. It was cheap. We were testing it." Police had information that was potentially helpful to the public health response to addiction. Sharfstein remarked, "You'd be surprised what other people know that's relevant, even within the city government."

In the current initiative between the Johns Hopkins Bloomberg School of Public Health and the Baltimore Police Department there is a recognition that bringing in others to look at police data may further department goals to reduce violence and enhance community trust. The Police Department does not typically disclose its data in that way, but for the purposes of this initiative, it has recognized the value of sharing data. According to Sharfstein, the police commissioner has said that the department does not want to do things that don't work and is counting on the Hopkins team to tell them if something is not working.

Sharing and Using Personal Health Data Collected by Individuals

Typically health data have been collected by researchers and by the health care delivery system. But more and more people are using fitness trackers and other personal health monitoring devices, while the number of health-related applications for smartphones and computers is increasing exponentially (a topic that is also explored in *The Tyranny of Evidence*, the opening chapter of this section). How should data collected by individuals and by third-party application providers be handled and what are the challenges attendant on their use?

There are many methodological and validity challenges associated with the collection and use of self-reported data, noted Sharfstein, quoting an NIH epidemiologist discussing a scenario of a million volunteers sharing their data, who said, "You don't get to suspend the rules of epidemiology when you have a cohort of volunteers . . . There's a science to it that maybe isn't as well developed as the enthusiasm about it."

The top public health priority is solid population-based data, such as exists in the health care system. For example, if data on all hospitalizations from asthma or all gunshot wounds are available, these can be mapped so that interventions can be developed. Such data can be collected at a population level in real time.

The methodological challenge with personal monitoring devices such as fitness bands, according to Sharfstein, is identifying the core outcomes being addressed. Then perhaps a fitness band, for example, may become a means to an end.

At the same time, how the individual actually uses a device—how properly, consistently, and rigorously—can significantly affect the integrity of the data, pointed out Damon Davis, MBA, director, Health Data Initiative, at the Office of the Chief Technology Officer in the Department of Health and Human Services. "The usability of some of these things is going to be extremely important as we move into a broader set of data sharing that comes from individual sources, clinical sources, federal sources, and special cohorts. More data is not always going to be better."

The generation and use of patient-reported data is still new, but expanding rapidly and likely to require something of a culture change as researchers, providers, and public health agencies consider data from non-delivery system sources.

Using Shared Data for Other Than the Original Purpose

Data collected for a health purpose may be relevant for other purposes, such as investigating Medicaid fraud or making referrals to social services. What are the implications of such use?

A health project should be about improving health, stressed Sharfstein. Eliminating Medicaid fraud is a worthy goal, but it requires another framework and handling by those charged with such investigations, such as the Attorney General's Medicaid Fraud Unit. "The framework of public health use of data should be about helping," he said.

On the other hand, there is a lot of interest in the use of predictive modeling to identify individuals at clinical risk (such as an elderly person with certain health conditions at risk for a fall or a patient on pain medication who may become addicted to opioids) and offer preventive services. But such efforts may also be viewed as meddling and intrusive.

Meshing clinical and social service data sets with the goal of identifying individuals who have both clinical and social service needs (for example, because they are unable to pay a heating bill), and then discussing needs with them, is not an easy process. Indeed, this can be "an incredibly challenging conversation to have," said Davis, "regardless of how altruistic your vision is for trying to marry up those two datasets: the clinical versus the social service needs."

Public health has the skills to get over that barrier, said Sharfstein, perhaps more so than a busy clinician's office. It is key to think through data use in such situations so as to prevent unintended consequences and ensure that the people attached to the data are receiving the benefits of data sharing.

Defining Ownership of Personal Health Data and Who Benefits (or Loses) from Its Use

Sharing of personal health data can be a sensitive topic, as the people whose data are being shared may have a range of concerns about the use of their data by others. The question then is: Who owns and gets to benefit from the use of personal health data?

Use of personal health data raises issues around health equity and race and class. Individuals may not trust researchers or a public health or social services system to handle their health data appropriately. They may be concerned that such data will be used against them—for example, to take their children away if they are seen as not able to provide housing. Or they may question why, if their data contributed to the development of a new medication or treatment, they should not benefit financially from that if there is money to be made from the innovation.

Sharfstein emphasized the importance of sharing personal health data for public and individual good. "We can really help people by sharing data," he said, noting that a thoughtful plan for data use can mitigate people's concerns. Yet, some may be unwilling to have their data shared and just drop out of the system.

The sharing of data—and not just data but the analysis, interpretation, and modeling that lead to knowledge—is a key piece in the scaffolding of a Culture of Health. Along with the traditional health care system, federal, state, and local governments; academic and public health researchers; police departments, housing authorities, substance abuse programs, and other public agencies; school districts; businesses; and other organizations and groups all have knowledge to contribute to the improvement of individual, community, and societal health.

At the same time the analysis and comingling of data on a scale never before possible is a cultural change that brings technological challenges and raises substantive concerns about data quality, privacy, and ownership that must be addressed with integrity in a way that appropriately balances individual and community interests. There is much to consider as researchers, policymakers, and practitioners take advantage of groundbreaking technological innovations and very large amounts of data to work together to build a Culture of Health that is equitable and inclusive.

7

The Importance of Community-Based Participatory Research

CHRISTOPHER GIBBONS, MD, MPH, CHIEF HEALTH INNOVATION
ADVISER, FEDERAL COMMUNICATIONS COMMISSION

CONSUELO H. WILKINS, MD, MSCI, EXECUTIVE DIRECTOR,
MEHARRY-VANDERBILT ALLIANCE

The call to engage local people in research that affects them is familiar to almost anyone who works at the intersection of community and scholarship. But answering that call is not a simple process. Every step—from the strategies used to involve residents, to decisions about how their input will be incorporated into study designs, to what gets left behind when researchers depart—can be challenging, complex, and sometimes controversial.

The challenges begin with terminology—researchers may refer to their work as community-based participatory research, community-informed research, community-led research, or citizen science, and assign different meanings to each phrase. Regardless of the definition, a full-tilt commitment to nontraditional approaches can be hampered by limited funding, long-held views about how research should be conducted, doubts about the rigor of alternative designs, and the sheer effort required to involve historically disenfranchised stakeholders.

Nonetheless, "community-based research" returns almost 74 million results in a Web search. There is growing recognition that empowerment is a crucial driver of the behavior changes that support a Culture of Health—and that to be empowered a community's voice must be heard in the design and implementation of studies that influence practice and policy.

But there is still no consensus on a set of interrelated questions: Just what does it mean to seek participation from the community? Who decides what questions are asked and who answers them? Who benefits from the end results?

Valuing the Community Contribution

Disadvantaged communities are not always understudied ones. Health researchers at Johns Hopkins University—which Christopher Gibbons describes bluntly
as "an elite academic institution located in an urban ghetto"—looked back at a
decade of scholarship and estimated that some 500 papers had been published
about the East Baltimore community that surrounds the medical center. And
yet, Gibbons said, "the community hasn't actually changed. It hasn't gotten any
better."

Findings like that give rise to the term *helicopter research*. "That's what the
population says we do," observed Gibbons. As skeptical residents see it, "you design your studies, you get your funding, you come in, drop down, involve me for
a little while, get your results, go back, get promoted, get rich, and go away." But
one result remains the same: "The community never changes."

The emerging emphasis on stakeholder engagement is intended to animate
new approaches. "The way we've done traditional health research within con-
fined laboratories is one way of doing research, but it is not the only way," said
Deborah Bae, MPA, MBA, a senior program officer at RWJF. "Increasingly, we
are finding a range of ways to do research that includes the participants from
whom we are getting information and data."

Whether the goal is to inform biomedicine or change behavior, the nuanced
and complicated process of community engagement can, at its best, bear succu-
lent fruit for those who nurture it.

More Than Window Dressing

When he first became involved in community-based research, Gibbons assumed
that his own racial identity would give him something of a free pass in communities of color. "I think I know something about black communities. I grew up in
a black home. When I started doing this community work years ago, I thought,
'oh great. I'm the black guy and I'm leading stuff and they're black people. This
is going to be good.'"

Instead, "I got killed over and over and over again because I just wasn't giving
them what they wanted."

Determined to confront his own assumptions, Gibbons and a study team
from Johns Hopkins committed themselves to a full partnership with local
people, embedding them into the research from its earliest stages. Rather than
define a question or hypothesis first, and then bring the community in to examine it, they approached local leaders and said, essentially, "We'd like to improve health; let's come together and see if this can be done."

A long and troubled town/gown history dogged the work—"we were afraid in the beginning that it would lead to bloodshed," said Gibbons, only partially in jest. But despite deep suspicions and a bitter past, 100 local people showed up for an initial meeting.

The level of interest continued, but the way forward remained slow and bumpy. Consensus on the context in which the research should occur was elusive, and no assumption went unchallenged: What is community? Who speaks for that community? Do we have the right people involved? As Gibbons cautions, "Just because you have a couple of colors at the table does not ensure that they are the right people."

Typical of the challenges was the notion of how community should be defined. Researchers routinely place a set of boundaries around their study population—defining it by ZIP code or police precinct or sociodemographics, for example. But local people have their own ideas about the reach of their community, and that discrepancy often led someone to complain, "You didn't get this person, you didn't get that part of the community."

There were also differing views on what data would be most valuable, how to collect and use data, and how best to cycle data back to research participants. "What people in the community consider data is very different from what we consider data," acknowledged Gibbons. "And if you're interpreting it without them, your interpretations will be different than if you give them the raw data and ask them what they think."

Step by painstaking step, Gibbons and his research time soldiered on to design and conduct a study that would be meaningful to everyone involved. Often, when they thought a set of issues had been resolved, another sensitive topic would arise to block any forward movement. At one point, local residents asked for some core shifts in the focus of the work, forcing Gibbons' team to think deeply about who was in charge. "If we had said 'no,' then who is really leading the research? Who is it really about?"

Harnessing the Power of Self-Determination

Community members have so much knowledge and expertise, but we don't empower them to use that.—Deborah Bae

Seeing local people as an asset to research, not a constituency to be mollified, can open the door to fuller partnerships. But the mind-set often lingers among scholars that community-based participatory research is a "diminution of expertise," warned Peter Levine, PhD, Lincoln Filene Professor of Citizenship and Public Affairs at Tufts University.

In fact, quite the opposite may be true. Because they have intimate knowledge of their own communities, local residents often know best how to improve health outcomes for themselves, their families, and their neighbors, and what kinds of programs and practices will drive better results on the ground.

A rich package of research examples from the field suggests a shift is in process. Putting residents at the front and center of information-gathering is one way forward, as seen in a community where young men were paid a living wage to survey their neighbors. In another example, residents came together to develop an asset map of food sources.

Local groups can also translate their own knowledge into action, as one did by bringing tai chi classes for seniors into a park, thereby transforming a location that had been inundated with drug use into a valued neighborhood amenity. Elsewhere, residents organized to promote backyard gardens, rather than community gardens, because their experiences had taught them that the latter were vulnerable to vandalism.

These approaches are part of a larger movement to let underserved communities lead, in partnership with funders, rather than act as passive recipients of grants that promote preconceived approaches. A commitment to self-determination—the process by which a community determines its own values and forms its own allegiances and governance—gives these actions a power that can last beyond their immediate goals.

Peer Learning

Another way to validate local expertise is to recognize its utility as a peer-to-peer educational tool. An example from India serves as a reminder that low-resource communities, both in the United States and abroad, are often authorities on "frugal innovations" that can be tested and shared.

Indian farmers had not been very responsive to government workers who were trying to help them improve their agricultural practices. But when farmers from their own communities used low-cost video technology to explain their successful techniques, the response improved dramatically. That kind of community-led education is equally suited to the United States, where locally made videos demonstrate a capacity to improve health knowledge and behavior related to diabetes, HIV, maternal health, and much else.

"It's about letting people who are leaders in a community speak directly to that community," said David Fleming, MD, vice president of global health at PATH, reflecting on the Indian experience. PATH focuses on health innovations worldwide. He continued, "We have a community asset model: most of the resources we need are already there. We need to do better building on assets we already have."

The power of a common background and shared experiences can also be embraced in research designed to understand local realities. Assigning interviewers who look like the people they are interviewing can increase the chance of a candid conversation, leading to actionable research results.

Making It Happen

Technology, new ways of thinking about hierarchy and expertise, and respect for ideas born and nurtured in the community have pushed citizen science forward, but the tools to spread it more widely are still being developed.

Obstacles of tradition, funding streams, and competitive pressures loom large, and academic worth continues to be measured primarily by publications in prestigious journals. "Most people who hold the reins of funding were not trained in this area, and so their ability to understand it, and therefore to value it" is limited, said Gibbons. "I've had several people tell me, 'look, you can't just do community-based research and expect to survive. You can't do that and get promoted.'"

Indeed, Gibbons went further to suggest that the "industry" of academia would be threatened if it were forced to substantially change the way it does business. Inertia favors the status quo, especially when so many scientists remain convinced that the capacity to create valid knowledge rests exclusively with them.

"We want evidence-based decisions, but we want the evidence-based decisions that we as scientists think are right, without really accounting for the values of the people we're working with," said Anna Hoover, PhD, MA, who co-directs the National Coordinating Center for the RWJF-funded program Systems for Action. "So the idea is if we can get them involved and we can get them the information, they'll do what we would do. And then we get mad when they don't."

What Hoover called a "discourse of deficiency" tends to undervalue grassroots contributions. Even where researchers are open to nontraditional strategies, many simply do not know how to engage community members, or do not recognize the imperative of involving them as equals. Consuelo Wilkins recalls, "When I got my master's in clinical investigation, there was not one hour, or even 15 minutes, devoted to 'how do you get input from community members and act on it?'"

Changing Perspectives

Despite these and other barriers, new models for conducting, disseminating, and rewarding research are of growing interest. The era of precision medicine, which by definition tailors prevention and treatment to individual variability in environment, lifestyle, and genes, requires scientists to engage more directly with their study subjects. A crop of peer-reviewed journals, like *Progress in Community Health Partnerships: Research, Education and Action*, have been launched to publicize local partnerships that approach research in novel ways in order to improve public health. Some universities are assigning greater value to community-oriented research or the willingness to share data more broadly (as described in the previous chapter, *The Secrecy Divide*) in their promotion and tenure decisions.

Social media, crowdsourcing, and health informatics also introduce powerful strategies for listening to, and learning from, the community. Patients Like Me (*patientslikeme.com*) is an online network that has grown to 400,000 patients who share data on symptom and treatment experiences. As its website proclaims, "That data helps you track how you're doing over time, helps the next person diagnosed learn what could work for them, and tells researchers what people really need so they can develop more effective treatments, faster."

The message of all that, said Gibbons, is that "if we continue to drag our feet, people will just go forward. The idea that people are waiting for science to catch up with them is a fallacy. African-Americans in East Baltimore and West Baltimore are not sitting around waiting for somebody at Johns Hopkins to tell them what to do. They're trying to figure it out on their own. Is that science? Of course. It's a type of science, but not the one that's valued over here."

What Researchers Need to Consider

Bring the Community In Early and Often

"Having community members on at the beginning to help refine your proposals and your protocol adds so much value as you think about all the other steps in the research process," said Wilkins. Local stakeholders who serve as co-principal investigators, research partners, advisory group participants, or in other capacities can influence hypotheses and study designs, guide recruitment, and ultimately contribute to outcomes that are relevant to the community.

Learn to Listen

At Vanderbilt University, a "community engagement studio" gives researchers a chance to learn from the population they expect to study. At one such convening, potential study participants recommended overhauling a recruitment flyer designed to attract African-American women and offered advice on how to recruit, where to post the flyers, and why having culturally congruent staff is essential. The result: recruitment increased by 78 percent, researchers met their accrual goals 16 months ahead of schedule, and there was no loss to follow-up.

Build Trust in Ways that Resonate

Resource-challenged communities that have been historically excluded from decision-making think differently about trust than do scholars in academic settings. Where researchers may consider competency, education, and funding as essential to collecting trustworthy results, "people who have been marginalized are concerned about safety and fairness," Wilkins explained. They are especially likely to worry about being randomized to treatment that may prove to be less effective or harmful, and often have to be persuaded that research results are valid.

Gaining the trust of stakeholders goes hand in hand with involving them in meaningful ways. Wilkins described a study in which local residents helped to assess the relationship between asthma and air quality in their own public housing community. "When you have people involved and they're actually helping to collect the data and they're thinking about what the outcomes might be, their investment in the process is certainly different. They're more likely not just to have confidence in the results, but to share them with others, and encourage other participation."

Structure a Fair Transaction

Framing the relationship between researchers and the community as transactional helps to raise up the issue of fairness. Research can place a burden on a community and researchers have an obligation to give back something of value as part of the exchange.

Money is one of the more delicate issues that can arise in this discussion. Paying research participants can be a contentious practice, and in some study designs it can distort or invalidate findings. But no one expects scientists and researchers to work without earning a salary, so there is an inherent imbalance in the assumptions that get made about rewards.

A classic example is the well-known story of the HeLa cells, the immortal cells culled from Henrietta Lacks, which enriched an industry and changed the world, but provided no gain to her impoverished family, which still lives in East

Baltimore. (For more information, see the book *The Immortal Life of Henrietta Lacks* by Rebecca Skloot.) There are not always easy ways to reward the contributions of study subjects, but the issue demands due consideration.

Return Results

Researchers seeking community participation are often asked by local people, "What do I get out of it?" The answers are not always straightforward or uniform—not everyone who participates in a study that collects genetic data will want the test results, for example. "We have to think about how we design a project that will be meaningful to them, that will give them something back, and that they'll want to participate in," emphasized Wilkins.

How Systems Need to Change

Build the Infrastructure for Community Research

A number of individual public and private sector initiatives have been developed to train scholars in some form of community-based research, and to grow the pool of researchers from communities of color. However, these have not been institutionalized or widely replicated in university settings, especially in the biomedical field.

A core recommendation of the National Academy of Medicine (formerly Institute of Medicine), in a report on its Clinical and Translational Science Awards program, is to "ensure community engagement in all phases of research." Broad commitments are needed to make that happen, said Wilkins. "It's critical that we think not just about single programs that are focused on community-engaged research, but about how the curricula in biomedical research need to change so that we have community engagement in all of them."

Training community health workers to design and conduct research is one pathway of interest. "There's a very strong opinion that basic research skills should be part of the preparation of community health workers," said Carl Rush, MRP, a public health policy specialist at the University of Texas School of Public Health, describing an emerging consensus on their scope of practice and skill requirements.

Honor "Program Building"

To counter the system that structures publishing as the primary way to advance an academic career, there should also be rewards for establishing enduring programs.

Harolyn Belcher, MD, MHS, director of the Center for Diversity in Public Health Leadership Training at the Kennedy Krieger Institute in Baltimore, engaged Head Start staff in parenting intervention studies so that actionable knowledge would be left behind once university researchers departed. "The work might generate only one or two articles because it is so labor intensive, but then you can say you're a program builder," she said.

Build Capacity for Action

Improving local conditions lies at the heart of community-based research. "Data is not valuable unless you've taken that data and actually done something with it involving the community," said Gibbons.

But he cautioned against a framework that said, in essence, communities should be empowered to fix their own problems. "We academics say that when we don't know what to do . . . Participatory action research gets me as an academic off the hook because I can say 'I've done the research, I gave it to the community, and if they can't do anything about it, it's their problem.'" The truth, Gibbons emphasized, is that neither researchers nor local people can implement solutions alone. "The only way something is going to happen is if we come together and work together and find solutions together."

Scale Smart

Find out what is working locally, and involve communities in bringing those models to scale. "We need micro experiments to feed into policy," said CMS's Karen Matsuoka. "Don't do broad, macro-level changes and then figure out that they don't work. Empowering communities is the way to move the needle."

Community-based research, however it is defined, does not replace traditional models of research entirely, but it surely enriches and supplements them. It offers a way to use data as a tool to drive action, and promotes a multidirectional flow of information that respects the unique skills and perspectives that all participants bring to the process.

Building the powerful, respectful partnerships that can make that happen is an iterative process. In East Baltimore, Gibbons and his team made a nonnegotiable commitment to work with anyone from the community who wanted to be involved, regardless of when in the process they surfaced. Often enough, that meant playing out the same discussion whenever someone new showed up at a meeting, sometimes to berate efforts that were already underway.

The first several times that happened, no one else in the room disputed the vocal contention that university researchers were, once again, exploiting local people. But then something shifted, recalled Gibbons. One night, a newcomer stood to make that familiar complaint, but this time someone else rose next to declare fiercely, "You don't know what's going on here. This is different."

It was a lightbulb moment, a powerful reminder that things can actually change. "It's long and it's hard, but that's the kind of stuff that keeps me in this every single day," Gibbons said. "If you learn how to work together effectively, more will happen than you could ever dream."

PART FOUR

CRITICAL PATHWAYS
FOR SYSTEMS CHANGE

If *Views on Understanding Culture, Experience, and Health* sharpened our understanding of the challenges we face as a society, and *Pursuing Knowledge with Purpose* told us what makes research effective, *Critical Pathways for Systems Change* offers reassurance that the work moves ahead even as we continue to learn. The growing recognition that the drivers of health need to be considered in a larger context seems to have reached an inflection point, with cross-cutting work underway at the level of family, health system, community, nation, and planet.

The concept of the commons is very much in evidence in these undertakings, as program planners and policymakers think broadly about what it takes to build a good society. Surely that must include nurturing children, and sparing them exposure to violence, topics explored in *Fostering Healthier Environments for Children and Families*. A sense of coming together is also evident in *Aligning Systems of Health and Health Care*, which looks at how providers can reach beyond the walls of their institutions to generate greater health within their communities.

Building Healthy Cities paints a picture of vibrant urban settings designed to work for all their residents while *Rethinking How We Police Communities* highlights the threads that tie law enforcement and policing together, and asks us to consider what we really mean when we talk about the need for security. The closing chapter, *Climate Change Through a Health Lens*, circles back to our obligations to generations yet to come, while putting the issue of planetary health squarely within the context of other health-building activities. This is a relatively new addition to RWJF's portfolio, allowing us to build on the long-standing efforts of so many others.

Coming together across disciplines is a core part of growing a movement, which is the force that powers a Culture of Health. Partnerships that thrive on mutual respect, and collaboration with unlikely partners who force us to move outside our silos, are among the core strategies outlined in the following chapters. While optimistically describing the co-benefits of a shared agenda, the work also recognizes that to progress, we must sometimes accept incremental improvements, not the wholesale transformation we might prefer. It also cautions us of the consequences if we fail to put vulnerable populations at the front and center of our commitments.

Fostering Healthier Environments for Children and Families

MAX CROWLEY, PHD, ASSISTANT PROFESSOR, HUMAN DEVELOPMENT
AND FAMILY STUDIES, COLLEGE OF HEALTH AND HUMAN DEVELOPMENT,
PENNSYLVANIA STATE UNIVERSITY

RON HASKINS, PHD, MAT, SENIOR FELLOW, ECONOMIC STUDIES,
AND CO-DIRECTOR, CENTER ON FAMILIES AND CHILDREN,
BROOKINGS INSTITUTION

EBONI HOWARD, PHD, MANAGING RESEARCHER, AMERICAN
INSTITUTES FOR RESEARCH

DEBRA L. NESS, MS, PRESIDENT, NATIONAL PARTNERSHIP
FOR WOMEN & FAMILIES

The Culture of Health begins with the family, a child's first and most important environmental context for development. The ecological circumstances of American families have undergone significant changes over the last four decades, with more mothers working full-time, a decline in marriage rates, and an increase in non-marital births. In light of changing family structures, what can be done to nurture the strengths of families and ensure that children develop well and grow into healthy, productive, and thriving adults?

The contributors to this chapter considered that question from many vantage points—examining a movement to change the culture of work, the effects of changing family structure, the long-term benefits of emotional self-regulation, and how to put what we know into the healthy development of young children. Together they offer a window into improving the policies and programs for child and family health.

We begin with a look at how changes in the culture of work can contribute to healthier families—and what it takes to make this happen. This is followed by a discussion of evolving family structure and its implications for the well-being of children.

Building a Movement for Healthier Families

The mission of the National Partnership for Women & Families (*www.national-partnership.org*), according to its president, Debra Ness, "is to create a society in which everybody can thrive and prosper and participate to the fullest extent of their abilities." In order to do that, said Ness, people must have economic security and access to good health and health care, and be able to care for themselves and their families—and all must have these to ensure an equitable society.

It was a desire for equity—equity for women and men in the workplace—that drove the thinking that led to the Family and Medical Leave Act of 1993.[1] Previously the National Partnership had devoted much effort to passing laws and establishing a legal infrastructure to support women's equality in the work setting, but "not a whole lot had changed because the stereotypes about women as caregivers and men as breadwinners were as alive and well as ever," said Ness.

So the question was raised: What can be done in the workplace to address the fact that working people also have family lives? The idea for the Family and Medical Leave Act was born, but not well-received. "People thought we were nuts," said Ness. "They said it was going to be the end of free enterprise as we know it."

It took a decade of hard work to finally bring the bill to President Bill Clinton's desk for his signature on February 5, 1993—one of his first acts as president. Twenty years later Clinton noted that he had received more thanks from citizens for the passage of the Family and Medical Leave Act than for any other single piece of legislation.

Since its passage, said Ness, the law has been used 200 million times by workers: "The most profound difference the [Family and Medical Leave Act] made is the change in the way we think about the workplace and what we expect now."

Pivotal Factors in Building the Movement

Ness described factors leading to the passage of the Family and Medical Leave Act that are key to building any movement:

---

[1] To find out more about FMLA, go to *www.dol.gov/whd/regs/statutes/fmla.htm.*

- *Having a vision that resonates with people in a very gut-level, emotional way.* When advocates shifted the conversation from the personal struggle of individual women to a family issue, they were able to create a vision that engaged many.
- *Building the broadest coalition possible.* Advocates brought together more than 300 groups representing women, children, labor, seniors, and advocates for health, disability, religion, and civil rights. Leveraging people with different strengths, constituencies, and relationships is essential.

  Catholic bishops signed on in the belief that if pregnant women knew they had a job to go back to they would be less likely to seek an abortion. Their endorsement was critical, said Ness. "If we hadn't had the Catholic bishops, we wouldn't have gotten that bipartisan support."
- *Telling real-life stories that help people understand how this will affect them.* Vice President Al Gore, on the floor of the Senate, told of being in the hospital with his young son who had been hit by a car and seeing parents who could not stay with their seriously ill children because they were afraid they might lose their job. His story was powerful and convincing.
- *Being committed for the long haul.* Despite steady work on an issue, progress may be hard to see, said Ness. "And then there are those catalytic moments when things catch fire." During the decade leading to the passage of the Act dozens of states passed similar laws. Eventually, the climate was right for passage at the federal level.

The movement was committed to *family* leave, rather than a narrow (but probably more easily passed) focus on maternity leave. The goal was to make full involvement in family life easier for men, while allowing women to participate fully in work life.

This experience underscores the culture shifts that are needed when building a movement for lasting social change. "You want to be able to change culture at the same time that you're trying to change policy. The two interact with each other and the journey is not a straight line and it's not an overnight thing," said Ness.

The Work Continues

Some 40 percent of American workers still do not have access to family and medical leave because they work for small organizations, work part-time, or are otherwise ineligible under the law. But Ness noted that conversation about work and family issues has intensified in the last two to three years—no accident, she said, since the coalition has stayed alive, growing through electronic communication and social media. Some good news:

- California, New Jersey, and Rhode Island have *paid* family and medical leave laws, and New York is very close to passing one.
- Five states and 28 local areas have paid sick days for their workers. Yet, 80 percent of low-wage workers have no paid sick days at all.

Family and medical leave has direct impacts on individual families and, more generally, contributes to a Culture of Health. Newborns are more likely to be breastfed, get checkups, and be immunized. Fathers are more involved in the care of their children. A sick child's hospital stay may be shortened by a parent's presence.

Workplace laws that help families also benefit employers and society as a whole, Ness pointed out. Workforce attachment increases and new mothers return to the same employer and are more likely to be employed and promoted and to earn higher wages. Employers save money by reduced employee turnover. Providing all workers with paid sick days would result in 1.3 million fewer emergency room visits annually, a societal savings of about $1.1 billion, according to Ness. She concludes, "The sky didn't fall, our economy didn't collapse, and, for the most part, employers have done fairly well."

Responding to Changing Family Structure

The last four decades have seen substantial changes in the composition of the American family—changes that have important implications for child and family health, according to Ron Haskins. Haskins identified two key trends:

- Marriage rates have declined steadily. Many fewer people get married now, with the exception of college-educated women, who are very likely to get and stay married and are unlikely to have children outside marriage—all of which gives their children "quite an advantage," noted Haskins.
- At the same time, non-marital birth rates have risen for every group. Now four out of 10 American children overall are born outside marriage, and the figures are higher among populations of color—a little more than seven of 10 black children and about four and a half out of 10 Hispanic children are not born to married parents. As a result, many more children are living with a single parent; of those, 85 percent live with a mother and 15 percent with a father.

What Difference Does This Make?

Three major consequences stand out:

- *Higher child poverty rates.* A child living in a single-parent family is five times more likely to live in poverty than a child in a married-couple family. And the "problem is getting worse, not better," said Haskins, adding that "this is part of the culture of families that has changed amazingly over the last four decades."
- *More income inequality.* The already large differences in income between single-parent and married-couple families are increasing.
- *Large, negative impacts on child development.* Compared with children living with married parents, children in single-parent families are:
  - Less likely to complete high school
  - More likely to get into trouble at school
  - More likely to get pregnant or to contribute to a pregnancy
  - More likely to be arrested.

Children living in single-parent families are also less healthy, said Haskins, and it is harder to reach out to single parents given their many obligations and time constraints, particularly if they are working, as public policy encourages.

How Have Policies Helped—and Not Helped?

The degree to which policy has successfully supported marriage varies quite a bit.

- While many people believe that there is a substantial tax disincentive to marriage, Haskins disagrees. For low-income couples the earned income tax credit[2] is actually a marriage booster. But more could be done to use tax policy to encourage marriage, he said, especially for couples with $25,000 to $30,000 in combined income.
- Welfare is a disincentive to marriage, as welfare benefits may be reduced for some couples when they marry, but that policy could be changed.
- Marriage education, a big program of the George W. Bush administration, has not worked well, according to Haskins. A strong, well-designed program might have an impact, but it is "nothing like an overall solution."
- Family and medical leave is important to do and needs more work, said Haskins, echoing Ness's discussion.

---

[2] The earned income tax credit (EITC) provides tax credits to low-income working families, primarily those with children. The income threshold at which EITC starts to phase out is higher for married couples than for unmarried individuals.

The best policy to help single mothers is the earned income tax credit, which has had mostly bipartisan support. "This is a huge achievement of American social policy," said Haskins. It was one of the factors that increased work participation when welfare reform was introduced during the Clinton administration, along with the requirements to receive welfare and the strong economy. "We've got millions of kids who are not in poverty by the combination of their mother working and public policy. We could do more of that. We could expand the work support system, especially earned income tax credit," he proposed.

Reducing Unplanned Pregnancies

Helping women control their fertility should be a number one goal of health policy and of overall American social policy.—Ron Haskins

Half of all pregnancies are unplanned, cutting across every demographic group, noted Debra Ness. "It's not a problem of just low-income women or women of color or young women."

A whole range of benefits would accrue, Haskins said: reduced poverty rates, better spacing of pregnancies, increased prenatal care, lower abortion rates, increased education completion rates for young women, and cost savings in government programs. Medicaid pays for contraception for low-income women and, while better implementation is needed, that "was a very wise thing," in Haskins' view.

Helping Single Mothers—and Fathers, Too

The single-parent trend cannot be reversed, Haskins believes. Perhaps marginal impacts can be made over 10 or 15 years, but a lot of children are growing up in single-parent families right now, and will continue to, "so we need to figure out good policies to help single mothers."

At the same time, Haskins acknowledges that "we've left men out of the equation to a substantial degree" and much better policies directed at men are needed. There is evidence that successful policies are possible, but Haskins stressed that "responsibility has to start with your financial responsibility to your children."

Session moderator Anthony Mingo, Sr.,[3] has both personal and professional experience with disadvantaged young men. Mingo believes that most men want to be involved in their children's lives and noted that there may be many reasons why a father in that environment is not engaged with his children. Mingo reported that

[3] Mingo is program coordinator of the Richmond (Va.) Family and Fatherhood Initiative. He moderated the lunch plenary session, along with Ness and Haskins.

fathers who participate in his program and begin to understand their significance and responsibility to their children tend to increase child support payments.

Reflections on Building a Movement for Today's Children and Families

Pay Attention to National Culture and History

It is well known that the United States lags behind many other developed Western countries in its family and workplace policies. Ness noted two key factors:

- American culture is "fiercely individualistic," fueled by a real "pull ourselves up by our bootstraps" mentality. This is important to keep in mind more broadly when working to build a Culture of Health in this country, she stressed.
- After World War II American men returned and women left the workforce and went back into the home. But in Europe the male population had been decimated and women continued to be needed in the workplace, so policies were created to make it possible for women to work outside the home.

Include Fathers in the Movement

Policy with regard to fathers seems to be "about the money," said audience member David Bishai, PhD, from Johns Hopkins Bloomberg School of Public Health. He asked whether there are ways to say to men, "We want your money *and* your time."

Haskins emphasized the importance of keeping the need for child support separate from the need for fathers to spend time with their children—one should not affect the other.

At the Richmond Family and Fatherhood Initiative, said Mingo, mothers stressed that the father's presence was most important to them, with money being second. They need help with their children and their children need to know their fathers. Mingo advocated for a less punitive and more engagement-focused approach that "pulls the guys out of the shadows, lets them know: 'you're not going to shirk this responsibility, but we're going to help you.'"

Consider Cultural Challenges That Impede Promotion of Family Health

Audience member Michael Rodriguez, MD, MPH, a family physician and professor at the David Geffen School of Medicine at UCLA, noted that cultural challenges, such as sexism and homophobia, get in the way of family health. He suggested that our culture can no longer tolerate abusive and nonrespectful discussions and references that are often driven by men. Instead, he said, "Men have to be more of an active player in the movement to eliminate violence against women, as well as in the movement to eliminate homophobia and sexism in all realms. When we do that, all members of our families will be much stronger."

Ness strongly agreed. "Culture change is really about changing people's hearts and minds, which then leads to changes in behavior and beliefs and eventually social norms. That is why the culture piece of change is just as important as the policy piece—if we do one without the other, we don't sustain the change."

Remain Optimistic About the Potential for Change

Social change, any kind of movement building, is messy. It doesn't lend itself to time lines and deliverables.—Debra Ness

Progress on social change "ebbs and flows," said Ness, so it is critical to ensure a strong infrastructure of "all stripes and types" of nongovernmental groups. "Government is very difficult to control. It's subject to political whims." She says that if we strive to keep the vision in the forefront, progress will happen.

In the current climate, coalition building can seem daunting, but as Haskins pointed out, "Things still happen. Some very important laws passed in the last several years." He also noted that Congress is "beginning to acquire a taste for evidence" and has funded states to test new ideas. Haskins believes passage of the proposed Family and Medical Insurance Leave Act[4] in some form is possible.

Evidence of economic impact, as well as constituent support, can help to change a conversation focused on government mandates and women's issues to one on how to move to a more competitive economy. "We're making progress. Behind the scenes, the conversation is changing," Ness predicts.

Self-Regulation as a Fundamental Social-Emotional Competency

Turning to the critical period of early childhood, researcher Max Crowley[5] emphasized emotional self-regulation as a core competency necessary for

---

[4] The Family and Medical Insurance Leave Act would provide workers in all companies regardless of size with partial income during up to 12 weeks of time off for pregnancy and childbirth, serious family medical issues, and so on. It would be funded by employee and employer payroll contributions.

[5] His colleagues are Damon Jones and Mark Greenberg of The Pennsylvania State University.

successful development into adulthood. He defined social-emotional competencies as "the fundamental ability to recognize and control our own emotions." A vast literature—from neurobiology to child development to sociology—provides evidence that children learn to recognize and control their emotions from supportive families, schools, and community cultures. And a growing literature demonstrates its importance.

What is lacking is the ability to consistently predict across the life span the effects of early childhood self-regulation and to understand the real value of being able to manage one's emotions. Crowley seeks to discover "what is that unique impact [of emotional self-regulation] and how does that fit into how we plan and build a Culture of Health."

Using "Big Science" to Answer "Big Questions"

This investigation of emotional self-regulation relies on a "big science mentality," bringing together an interdisciplinary group of experts in economics, psychology, sociology, and public finance to think about and answer questions about its unique value.

The group has undertaken an integrative data analysis of multiple longitudinal samples—"deep data sets" with annual assessments over decades. The cohorts are relatively small but include hundreds of baseline measures extending well beyond typical data sets. These include, said Crowley, "deep, consistent, thoughtful psychometrically valid measurement around emotional self-regulation in early childhood," as well as demographics; family structure; observations of home, community, and other environmental factors; and genetic and biological data.

Assembling an "Integrated Data Set"

The team combined the results of six longitudinal samples, following a total of more than 3,300 individuals for over three decades. This "integrated data set" represents more than $50 million in public research support to build the individual data sets and is "a national resource for answering these big questions," said Crowley.

The approach is multi-method, drawing on econometrics, statistics, machine learning, and engineering. Understanding that no one method is perfect, the hope is that using complementary methods will increase confidence about defining the value of social-emotional competencies.

The children in the samples were assessed for emotional self-regulation at age 6. Based on these assessments researchers were able to predict whether or not the children would later graduate from high school, be employed, be arrested by age 25, and need substance abuse treatment. "It replicates what we already knew to some extent: that this is a very important construct and skill in early life," said Crowley.

After applying the multi-method approach with increasingly rigorous methods, researchers found that the magnitude of the effect was lower than predicted, due to characteristics known to predict these outcomes (e.g., demographics, cognitive factors, family structure) and to health, biological, and other factors.

The researchers found that they could continue to significantly predict outcomes through these methods, but also that the magnitude of effects was consistent across the methods, increasing confidence that the estimates related to emotional self-regulation are stable and can be used for planning purposes.

Improving Outcomes Through Emotional Self-Regulation

If average self-regulation for 100 children increased from the 50th percentile to the 84th percentile, researchers would expect approximately: 5 more high school graduates; 3 more employed individuals; and 5 individuals not arrested who likely would have been.

From a fiscal perspective, this increase in average self-regulation would lead to savings of between $8,000 and $12,000 per youth, based on reduced criminal justice and Medicaid and Medicare costs and increased tax revenue. Crowley concludes, "[Emotional self-regulation] has clear value for children on outcomes not only important to the individual, but also to society, our culture, and how we live our lives—and they're also eminently monetizable."

Current effectiveness for effective social-emotional learning programs falls within a range of 0.2 to 0.4, said Crowley, citing a meta-analysis of 250 programs by Joseph Durlak, PhD,[6] and colleagues. Average cost to deliver these programs varies between $50 and $900 per child. The benefit to individuals and to society, if program strength could be increased without a large increase in cost, could be significant. The multidisciplinary research group proposed four ways to do that:

- *Continue to add new data.* This requires identifying samples, not publicly available, from researchers studying these issues for decades.
- *Enhance the outcome estimates,* moving beyond current fiscal projections to determining the direct impact on public budgets.
- *Design programs that move beyond a limited range of effects.* "There are many programs available, but no one has quite broken out of the pack in developing either a new kind of approach or a new type of curriculum," said Crowley.

[6] Durlak is professor emeritus of psychology at Loyola University Chicago and a consultant to CASEL, the Collaborative for Academic, Social, and Emotional Learning.

- *Focus on translating the evidence*. While translation of evidence in academic domains is strong, said Crowley, "we don't always do such a good job of thinking about these social-emotional elements."

Zeroing In on Methodology

Audience discussion elevated issues related to making the best use of the most data.

The Value of Multiple Methods

This is a "team science effort," as Crowley describes it, with a lot of back-and-forth to determine the standard of evidence for decision-making. The researchers have used, and continue to use, a variety of methods to look at the findings. For example, many samples included randomized controlled trials of early childhood programs that had significant effects on emotional self-regulation. The researchers leveraged the randomized design to do causal mediation analyses. Other contexts, with different designs and predictors, called for more naturalistic approaches.

As different models are developed researchers continue to look at the consistency of the outcome estimates. "Where we see consistency, we have greater confidence," said Crowley. "Where we don't see consistency, there may be factors that we're not including." Researchers seek to include additional data, for example, to increase sample sizes for small populations such as Native Americans.

Incorporating Real-Time Data for More Immediate Use

This is where being able to map directly onto administrative records is important and "where a lot of the opportunity is," said Crowley. It may be possible (and easier) to follow administrative data for decades, rather than do hours-long annual individual surveys. That would be "very exciting."

Using Predictive Models in Legislative Decision-Making

Legislative decisions about financing programs are being made based, at least in part, on the predictions of these models. "They're being used to set priorities, whether we agree with them or not," said Crowley. That makes their rigor and validity critical. Otherwise, in the push to do something, legislated programs will lack strong evidence. In addition, states are using models to make spending decisions that do not include social-emotional competency in the projections.

Integrating Social and Emotional Factors into Studying Child Health

The cross-sectional data sets can contribute to understanding the epidemiology of social-emotional health and other factors, said Crowley. He cited Canadian efforts to map social-emotional functioning at a neighborhood level. This is valuable for planning and offers potential to introduce interventions based on neighborhood results.

Putting What We Know into Practice

A wealth of scientific information about what matters for young children (from the prenatal period through age 5) is available from a range of disciplines, according to Eboni Howard, who brings 25 years of experience in child and family research to the conversation.

Understanding brain development has greatly expanded during Howard's career. Within the first three years of life the amount of brain growth is "incredible," she said. The brain of a newborn infant is about 25 percent the size of an adult brain. By age 3 the brain has grown to about 80 percent. A vast amount of activity is going on in the brain of the young child as neural connections are created and pruned. As Howard's research confirms, "We know that early experiences serve as a foundation for later learning, behavior, and health."

We also know that resources matter—and many children do not have the access to opportunities and resources needed to create a strong foundation for the future. A weak foundation makes it harder to develop skills and build health. "Skills beget skills," Howard emphasized. "Circuits build upon circuits. Early life experiences are going to affect later life experiences."

While we know that everyday experiences and resources both matter, there are great differences between knowing that and the reality of the lives of many children and families. Such children start life with disparities that continue through the life course.

How Do We Put What We Know into Practice?

Howard noted four major groupings of programs and services related to young children:

- **Early childhood education and care programs**, such as infant and toddler care, child-care centers, and preschool. While evidence suggests positive impacts from these programs, many questions remain about how to replicate them in broader populations.

- *Home visitation and parent support programs.* Some studies offer strong evidence of the positive impact of some home visitation programs, but different outcomes are found upon replication. Parent support programs receive a lot of anecdotal endorsement, but when scientific rigor is applied the evidence varies. In addition, methodological flaws limit the ability of these studies to determine what is causing the changes that do occur.
- *Family income and support programs,* such as WIC, earned income tax credit, family and medical leave, etc. Evidence of an impact on disparities and later child development and life success is unavailable. And disparities in who actually can use programs such as family and medical leave are significant, as Ness discussed earlier.
- *Pediatric screening, child abuse prevention, and early intervention programs,* which identify potential developmental needs and treatment for young children. There is "more theory and anecdote—a sense that this is right to do—than there is empirical evidence that such screeners are actually making a difference when it relates to equity and disparities," said Howard.

While many programs are available, not all are backed by solid evidence of the hoped-for impact for young children and their families, nor are they consistent with the resources and opportunities that are actually available. Ideally, we would use the knowledge we have to develop evidence-based interventions that can remedy inequality.

How Can Policy Help Parents Ensure Children Enter School Healthy and Prepared to Learn?

Many things may be suggested to parents as important for their children's health and readiness to learn—healthy cooking, reading to a child, developing household routines, to mention just a few. But in recommending actions to parents it is key to keep in mind that "there are families who just don't have enough and they're living in communities that don't have enough," said Howard. "How can I tell parents to do something when they're in this system that doesn't give them the opportunities to implement what I may want to share with them?"

Legislators don't want to hear about "opportunity gaps"—they must be given something tangible to support. As an example, Howard mentioned tax breaks to companies that establish supermarkets in neighborhoods lacking such facilities. "Then you can provide parent programs on healthy choices, because now they can access those healthy choices."

At the same time, Howard noted the broader impact of having business investment right in the neighborhood. It means, she said, that "those communities and those families feel like they matter. They're no longer being ignored. And that psychologically means a lot to parents for their kids." This can change the whole community psychology and bring in more resources.

Asked what young children need to ensure that they are healthy and safe and grow into productive adults, audience members offered many answers: love, parents, nurturing relationships, attention, stable housing, supportive schools, proper nutrition, and safe environments. Howard stressed the need to think about how to translate these ideas into actions and noted that what they mean will be rooted in different perspectives and belief structures: "The meaning is in our culture. The challenge is understanding our beliefs, values, and behaviors, and how they fit or not fit into what we think matters most for children."

It is a messy process, said Howard, but the resources and knowledge are there. "It's time now to take the next steps for action."

9

Aligning Systems of Health and Health Care

MANIK BHAT, CO-FOUNDER AND CEO, HEALTHIFY

SHERRY GLIED, PHD, MA, DEAN, ROBERT F. WAGNER GRADUATE
SCHOOL OF PUBLIC SERVICE, NEW YORK UNIVERSITY, AND FORMER
ASSISTANT SECRETARY FOR PLANNING AND EVALUATION, DEPARTMENT
OF HEALTH AND HUMAN SERVICES

MANMEET KAUR, FOUNDER AND EXECUTIVE DIRECTOR, CITY
HEALTH WORKS

ROCCO PERLA, PRESIDENT, HEALTH LEADS, AND FORMER SENIOR
LEADER, CENTERS FOR MEDICARE & MEDICAID SERVICES

Can we build health and health care systems where physicians write prescriptions for food and heat for their patients in need? Where software systems align health care and community services to address social determinants of health in a highly reliable way? Where an innovative delivery system uses community-based or professional coaches and navigators to bridge the gap between health and health care in patients?

More than 70 years after the World Health Organization (WHO) defined health as "a state of complete physical, mental, and social well-being, and not merely the absence of disease or infirmity," programs like these are actually being tested in communities across the country to create a long-sought alignment and integration between health and health care. Embracing the WHO's decades-old definition of health, this growing Culture of Health landscape promotes a core principle that social determinants of health must be addressed by integrating multiple layers of care with social services and community resources.

But how, exactly, does this bifurcated system of health and health care successfully align and integrate? How can the two sectors collaborate in ways that address micro changes like prescriptions for food alongside macro objectives that exist in health care, such as achieving true population health? How can a portion of the $3 trillion this country currently spends on health care be integrated into health-building services and programs that impact the social determinants of health? We know that these account for more than 60 percent of the modifiable factors influencing health outcomes and cost, so we are paying for the lack of alignment right now.

The four contributors to this chapter address these questions and argue that aligning and integrating clinical health care and health-building programs is essential to accelerate Culture of Health objectives. By sharing examples of delivery system innovations, they show how these two sectors can successfully collaborate and how this alignment can be measured and improved.

The Intersection of Health and Health Care

As an economist, Sherry Glied has spent her career doing research and creating policy on micro changes and their impact on health—"believing that we can make a difference with small incremental advances in policy, both in helping those in need and reducing poverty and perhaps inequality as well." And when it comes to the intersection of health and health care, Glied allowed that "micro approaches to this can actually also fit into macro thinking."

A Bifurcated System and Why It Exists

Glied defined the health-building sector as made up of nonmedical determinants of health and the socioeconomic determinants of health like housing, the built environment, and income; she defined health care as the clinical care sector, one that includes health care institutions that both prevent and treat illnesses. "It's obvious that we will always need both of those things. We will never get rid of the clinical care sector by building up the Culture of Health. The health-building sector can't do appendectomies, and hospitals are pretty lousy at paving sidewalks. We'll always have this bifurcated system."

Glied then argued that this bifurcated system forces individuals within both health and health care to think about "how we can make these two sectors collaborate in ways that address both micro changes and the macro concerns that we have."

Historically, she pointed out, the general link between the health-building sector and health outcomes is not new. Think about the social reform photography of New York journalist Jacob Riis in the late 1890s. Through photographs that documented the living and working conditions of the poor—especially inside tenement housing—Riis made the point that the health and well-being of impoverished families could be improved through better housing, adequate lighting and sanitation, and parks and playgrounds. Early laws related to public health were mostly written on the basis that improving housing, food, and even milk delivery would improve health.

"So we actually started this game by thinking about the non-health sector from a Culture of Health perspective," Glied said. "Today, though, we have laws and funding in all of these health-building areas, but there's no reason really to believe that these resources are being used in ways that optimally improve health or are based on scientific evidence. There's definitely lots of space for us to think about these policies and funding streams in new ways."

Overspending for Clinical Care, Underspending on Health-Building

To begin her discussion on funding streams and policies, Glied acknowledged the costs: "We spend $3 trillion on clinical care, substantially more per capita than any other country. So we spend a ridiculous amount of money on medical care. And we significantly underspend our peer countries on health-building activities."

According to Glied, overspending on clinical care and underspending on health building has helped create the following scenarios:

- "Our health-building safety net is crummy compared to many other countries while we spend a lot of money on clinical care."
- "Our health outcomes on average, and even among people near the top of the distribution, are poor."
- "We have growing inequality in income. There are communities of persistent and extreme poverty that are in truly dire situations."

These facts generate policy questions about a funding stream that skews to health care. Consider:

- How, ideally, should spending be allocated across sectors? How should the health-building sector and the clinical sector share in the funding?
- Who should get the checks? In a system that spends $3 trillion a year, should the clinical system get the money and buy services from the health-building sector? Or should the health-building sector get the money and buy services

from the clinical sector? "And if it's something else, what can we do to enhance those collaborations?"

- Is the answer to take that $3 trillion and give it to everyone else? To take it out of the hospital and put it back in the community? "It's a wonderful idea, but pragmatically challenging," Glied noted. "It's not how the clinical care system *really* works." Even more important, perhaps, Glied believes it's not how the system *should* work. She argued that the focus of various elements within the health-building sector should not be entirely on health outcomes. For instance, she said the housing sector should not focus entirely on whether it improves people's health, and the same should be said for our education system, too. She elaborates, "We want our children to learn history, to learn art, even if it does nothing at all for their health. So we have to be very careful not to be overly broad in this."

A Dangerous Path: Focusing on One Sector

Glied argued forcefully that all health-related dollars should not go entirely to the clinical care system, which would then be in a position to buy the non-health system services and fold health-building into clinical care operations. Calling this a "dangerous path," she likened this scenario to some of the most memorable scenes from the rock musical horror comedy film, *Little Shop of Horrors:* "Like Audrey II—*'Feed me! Feed me!'*—if the clinical care system sees money, they're incredibly politically adept at getting this money." All joking aside, she said, the real danger is actually three-fold:

- **If the clinical care system is allowed to determine the focus of the health-building sector, it will choose a small number of high-cost individuals and provide them with resources, a practice called "hot spotting."** With rare exceptions, Glied is opposed to this practice. "The kinds of problems we're talking about here, both in the micro and macro sense, are about communities. And most people in communities don't need clinical care right now. So if we move the responsibilities for these things into the clinical care sector, we're going to be focusing mainly on people who are already having problems. That could actually work to the detriment of our communities."
- **Most health-building programs do not save clinical costs.** "This is a point we've dealt with for many years in the prevention world. Most housing programs, improving housing, will not save money in the medical care sector. Improving education will not save money in the medical sector, at least not in the short run that we can measure. We've been down this road in prevention, in behavioral health, in a number of other places, and we know that most

programs do not save clinical care costs. But they do a lot of good. We need to be very, very careful that we don't focus too much on the possibility of saving money."

- **On the political side, there are also risks. Though some dedicated clinicians are focused on community and public health, on the whole the interest of the clinical care system is not on equity.** "By contrast, many of the health-building sectors are really focused directly on inequality and on the needs of those communities," Glied said.

"While I think there is a potential for the clinical care sector to take a large role here," Glied concluded, "there are real dangers in moving in that direction."

A Better Approach to Alignment: Collaboration

So how should this dual system work? How do you align two segments that could potentially compete for a pool of health and health care dollars? Glied called for an "explicit and deliberate approach" that focuses on collaborations to promote incremental or micro changes that will impact social determinants. She pointed out that this collaborative approach is grounded in four principles:

1. **A collaborative approach respects and maintains responsibility for an activity within the sector that is experienced in conducting that activity.** For instance, she said, the housing sector "is really good at housing and the clinical care sector is really good at clinical care. There are reasons economics says the division of labor is the source of the wealth of nations, and I believe that very profoundly. Let's have the people who know how to do something be the ones responsible for doing it."
2. **A collaborative approach designs policies with explicit goals that incorporate, but are not limited to, health outcomes, so that the health-building sector gets credit for when it improves health outcomes.**
3. **A collaborative approach routinely monitors and assesses progress toward its goals.** One such monitoring and assessment approach, said Glied, is "very old-fashioned: cost-benefit and cost-effectiveness analysis." Glied was quite passionate about this collaboration principle, pointing out that it belies a misconception about why putting money into the health-building sector is a good idea: prevention may not be *cost-saving*, but it is most often *cost-effective*. For instance, she said, it is much better to prevent a heart attack through having a blood pressure-controlling diet, than to treat it ex post. But if prevention programs seek to improve the diets of a population through interventions, it often costs more than the treatment would for the few people who will have

heart attacks. This reality often creates really targeted programs for the most at-risk individuals, "but that is the antithesis of community building." She clarifies, "So does that mean we shouldn't improve people's diets? Of course not. If you prevent the heart attack, you don't have the heart attack. And that is more important, I think, or at least as important, as the cost savings you get from it."

As a prime example of why to use a cost-benefit and cost-effectiveness analysis, Glied pointed to a national program called Housing First (*www.endhomelessness.org*), which helps provide permanent housing as soon as possible to people experiencing homelessness. The program has modest savings in clinical costs, Glied noted, so those only concerned about whether it saves money for the health care system would probably not fund it. "But it gives people housing, and housing has enormous benefits for people above and beyond the clinical benefits. You don't want programs like this to be measured entirely on the health side, and cost-benefit analysis and cost-effectiveness analysis are one tool in that way."

4. **A collaborative approach makes both sectors aware of the other sector's agenda, and uses evidence-based research and analysis to inform and advance those agendas.** To illustrate this point, Glied pointed to New York University's Policies for Action Research Hub, a RWJF-funded initiative that is one of five university-based hubs around the country designed to identify evidence-based social policies and develop metrics to implement these polices to improve health outcomes, while also linking data from non-health policy sectors like housing and transportation to data on health outcomes.[1]

As the leader of NYU's research hub, Glied oversees two research projects on the causal effects of housing and transportation on health. How does improving the quality of housing change health outcomes? How does transportation access affect health outcomes?

These studies, Glied noted, will ideally help create ways to measure what she calls "housing-sensitive" or "transportation-sensitive" conditions that impact health, a category akin to the "ambulatory-sensitive" conditions that are already tracked in hospital emergency room visits and admission. This hospital measure was developed 30 years ago by Glied's NYU colleague John Billings, PhD, professor of health policy and public service, who is widely known for his analysis of patterns of hospital admissions and emergency

[1] Policies for Action (P4A) is a RWJF research program administrated through the National Coordinating Center at the Urban Institute in collaboration with five research hubs at New York University, Temple University, The University of Illinois at Chicago together with Washington University at St. Louis, the University of Michigan, and the Urban Institute. For more information: *www.policiesforaction.org*.

room visits in vulnerable populations. It helps explain the links between access or a lack of access to primary care and hospital visits.

One of the goals of NYU's research hub is to develop a measure of housing or transportation that is similar to the measure of ambulatory-sensitive conditions. For instance, said Glied, "What are housing-sensitive conditions? For what kinds of conditions are people more likely to show up in the emergency room that are linked to the kind of housing that they live in? If we can come up with measures that actually have to do with housing, we can have housing authorities put 'health' on its dashboard. In New York City, the housing authority has 18 measures on its dashboard. None of them have anything to do with health."

Delivery System Innovations in a Fragmented System

When it comes to health and health care, delivery system innovations show how these two sectors can not only collaborate but also begin to measure this alignment. During a separate roundtable discussion that focused on delivery system transformation, presentations about three innovations—Healthify, City Health Works, and Health Leads—helped illustrate Glied's theory that micro approaches "can actually fit into macro thinking" when it comes to the intersection of health and health care.

These three initiatives, all recently supported by grants from RWJF, present opportunities to help communities manage their social determinants of health while promoting better health.

Healthify

We don't yet have enough data to claim that an approach leads to better health outcomes. Until we get that data, it will be difficult to have investment that leads to change in community.—Manik Bhat

The first message on Healthify's website reflects the touchstone of a Culture of Health: "There is more to health than health care." Billed as a user-friendly software solution, Healthify helps health care and community services address social determinants of health by working collaboratively. It provides services and Web technology to organizations like managed care plans and ACOs to find community services, connect patients to resources, screen for social needs, automate referrals, and track the progress in addressing social determinants.

Healthify uses the platform with health care clients that have over 5,000 staff in 25 states, conducting over 150,000 searches for services for people in need.

Led by co-founder and CEO Manik Bhat, Healthify recognizes that many communities have too many of some services and too few of others. "We see gaps between the needs and the service density in a region all the time," said Bhat, who started the company in 2013 in New York City. Health systems and hospitals "know they need to refer to these services more effectively." With data from 25 states now available, "we can get a pretty accurate assessment of gaps in communities. That information can be extrapolated more broadly to other communities. What we don't know yet is how different agencies run at the local level. That's going to change and vary widely. Knowing the supply and demand of needs and referrals can change how we approach the social services sector and how we invest there."[2]

In 2016, Healthify received pilot funding from RWJF's *Technology for Healthy Communities* program to partner with ACCESSHealth in Spartanburg, S.C. Together the two organizations will deploy a community resource platform to collect information on social and behavioral health needs and help provide community interventions.

City Health Works

City Health Works provides health coaching and care coordination for patients with chronic illnesses that helps bridge the gap between the doctor's office and the patients' everyday lives.

The organization shifts the center of health care from hospitals to the places where people live, work, play, and age, targeting populations who struggle with multiple chronic illnesses such as diabetes, hypertension, and asthma, along with stressors such as poverty and isolation. Founded in 2012 in New York by Manmeet Kaur, the organization partners with ambulatory care practices to give patients a system of health coaching and care coordination. The goals of City Health Works are two-fold: (1) helping health care practices more effectively manage the care of this high-need, high-cost population; and (2) helping patients gain confidence, through personal coaching and one-on-one conversations about medications, diets, and exercise, to take realistic steps that help them lead healthier lives and communicate more effectively with their doctors. "It will be game-changing, once we have a shared care plan that everyone can see. It

---

[2] Additional information about Healthify obtained from *Using Social Determinants of Health Data to Improve Health Care and Health: A Learning Report* published by the Robert Wood Johnson Foundation, May 2, 2016.

would reduce the confusion and fragmentation across the health care system and social sector," Kaur enthuses.

In 2015, RWJF approved a two-year grant to support City Health Works' effort to move from a pilot phase to a sustainable business model.

Health Leads

> *The health care landscape is littered with innovative ideas and new delivery and payment models. But if they don't come together in a systematic way— if they don't talk to each other—the result will be greater fragmentation, not less.*—Rocco Perla

Right now the health system needs the capacity to integrate social needs at scale—it's not just technology, but knowledge about scope of service and clinical workflows, tools and strategies that support high-quality implementation. These include screening tools based on validated instruments that have been tested in the field, and data that drive an understanding of which approaches to connect patients to resources work best under different conditions and which resources in a community are the most effective at meeting the needs of patients and families.

The Boston-based Health Leads has partnered with leading health care organizations across the United States for over 20 years to help them connect patients to community-based resources, ranging from food to transportation to health care benefits. In these two decades, the conversation in the health care sector has clearly moved from "should" social determinants of health be addressed to "how," noted Health Leads' president Rocco Perla, who joined the organization in 2016 after four years as a senior official at the Centers for Medicare & Medicaid Services.

Health Leads partners with health care organizations to enable physicians and other providers to prescribe food, heat, and other basic resources that patients need to be healthy. Patients then take these prescriptions to a Health Leads desk in the clinic waiting rooms, where trained advocates help them access community resources and public benefits. In this relationship model, advocates become "guests" in the lives of the patients they serve and guide them through the complex resource landscape.

Health Leads also enables health care organizations to track their social needs data through its Health Leads Reach™ platform. Risk factors like cholesterol and blood pressure improve when the full complement of resource needs are met, as does the system's overall ability to meet the needs of its patients.

In 2014, Health Leads received a multiyear, $16 million grant from RWJF to provide leadership to health systems and community health centers looking to address and achieve deep integration of patients' social needs.[3] In 2016, Health Leads launched the first in a series of toolkits to help health systems and clinicians screen for social needs and integrate social needs interventions into medical care. [4] Building this capacity across the health care sector is critical in 2017, as new initiatives go into effect that will require screening thousands to millions of patients for unmet social needs.[5] Achieving this step throughout the health care sector is critical to increasing the chances the model will succeed in improving care and reducing cost.

Reflections on Policy and Practice

In separate discussions with audience members, Glied, Bhat, Kaur, and Perla reflected on the policy and practice challenges they face when it comes to health and health care alignment.

Questions from multiple audience members after Glied's presentation zeroed in immediately to the heart of the matter:

- **Should we be thinking about *a* system as opposed to a bifurcated system? Who are the stakeholders engaged in this conversation?** Steven Woolf, PhD, director of the Center on Society and Health at Virginia Commonwealth University, pointed out that while there is a lot of money to leverage in the health care system, other sectors have a lot of resources and a "shared interest in making these investment. So it's really not just about the health and health care sectors. It's about bringing those different stakeholders to the table and coming up with an alignment of incentives."
- **What is the role of the Culture of Health in promoting well-being and recognizing the emotional determinants of health?** Christina D. Bethell, PhD, director of the Child and Adolescent Health Measurement Initiative at Johns Hopkins University, questioned where social and emotional determinants of health fit in: "This meeting has created an unstoppable force to bridge health and health care, especially by addressing the social determinants of health. But what about addressing the social and emotional determinants of health? Where do they fit in this?"

---

[3] For more information, search for "Health Leads" on *www.rwjf.org.*

[4] Read Health Leads' press release about the first toolkit here: *www.prnewswire.com/news-releases/ health-leads-screening-toolkit-equips-providers-to-take-first-step-in-addressing-patients-unmet-social-needs-300298185.html.*

[5] Recent policy efforts to address social needs alongside medical care include CMS's Accountable Health Communities and Comprehensive Primary Care Plus initiatives.

- **Where should funding come from?** Dr. Kevin G. Volpp, the founding director of the Center for Health Incentives and Behavioral Economics at the Leonard Davis Institute of Health Economics at the University of Pennsylvania, cautioned that while some health providers might appreciate that smoking and physical activity concerns are in their domain, "it would be the rare health care CEO who would appreciate that housing and education, some of the more important social determinants of health, are also in their domain. How do you overcome that?"

Glied agreed with both Woolf and Bethell that the Culture of Health is about "bringing stakeholders around the table." She also insisted that emotional well-being could not be overlooked. And while some health care money is already streaming into community development (for instance, Children's Hospital in Philadelphia is an anchor institution helping to build affordable housing while Medicaid dollars in New York City are going into its housing system), Glied agreed with Volpp that it would be very difficult to create a payment reform system requiring hospital CEOs to invest in housing or local education systems.

The three delivery system innovation panelists (from Healthify, City Health Works, and Health Leads) described an array of challenges—ranging from a lack of data and the struggle to understand which interventions work to navigating a fragmented landscape without coordinated reimbursement systems or full scale. Audience members peppered them with questions: How could these organizations address social determinants before people ended up in clinics? How could they translate data into more meaningful change? Should other service models be considered?

There were no easy answers. Feedback collection, for instance, continues to be a challenge at Healthify, which has tried to get feedback about social services from its clients (staff at managed care plans and integrated health care delivery networks) and the patients who are being referred for services; so far, this hasn't worked well. Though Healthify's system allows care managers and community health workers to rate services and comment on them, too few care managers and community health workers submit ratings and comments to make the data useful. To get feedback from patients, Healthify developed a texting system in which the person receives a text message with an option to message back. While Bhat believes that texting could still be a great way to get feedback from patients in certain communities, Healthify is looking at other ways to get feedback on services.[6]

---

[6] Additional information about Healthify obtained from *Using Social Determinants of Health Data to Improve Health Care and Health: A Learning Report* published by the Robert Wood Johnson Foundation, May 2, 2016.

Perla noted that rigorous and systematic follow-up with patients via the right mix of human and technological assets, along with clear definitions of what it means to successfully connect a patient to a resource, is the only way to ensure a high-quality resource database over time and to understand the effectiveness of the resource landscape. According to Perla, Health Leads' goal isn't to simply identify all the resources in an area, but to identify the ones that deliver results for patients and families and, therefore, for health care institutions. For instance, Health Leads' national data demonstrate that just 1 percent of the community resources in a given area drive 50 percent of successful outcomes, while 10 percent of resources drive 90 percent of successful connections. This example of a "narrow network" illuminates specific opportunities for targeted investment and collaboration across the health and social services.

To encourage community participation and help patients address social determinant issues before being referred to clinics, both City Health Works' Kaur and Healthify's Bhat noted that they recommend that their clients hire people from local communities to serve as health coaches and community health staff. Likewise, Health Leads arms health care institutions with the tools, technology, screening protocols, data, and analytics to deploy community health workers and others to work side by side with patients to access existing community resources. "When you hire someone from their community, that initial trust is already there," said Bhat.

One audience participant noted that while it's "great that we in health care are now identifying that this family doesn't have food and this one doesn't have housing," what happens when there are no more housing vouchers? When heating vouchers are gone? How do you address these broader system issues?

Bhat acknowledged that while there are resource gaps and capacity issues everywhere, collecting information long term to identify these needs and adopting a "very long trajectory" will one day help address the current constraint of "resources just not being there." Perla noted that while resource gaps can be problematic, the challenge is often one of information asymmetry and coordination of unmet needs with available resources. He shared an example from Contra Costa Regional Medical Center in California, where 60 percent of patients in one clinic reported not having enough food to last to the end of the month, while at the same time 40 percent of the CalFresh (food stamps) benefits in California go unclaimed. "Today, our health care system operates from an understanding of patients' social needs reminiscent of the sector before the Dartmouth Atlas and Framingham Heart Study illuminated flawed assumptions about the health of the population and geographic variation in cost, quality, and utilization. Until health systems commit to collecting social needs and resource connection data at scale, the Triple Aim will go unrealized," he concluded.

In closing, Glied allowed that measuring health alignment and collaboration through policy analysis is "as boring and wonky and micro as it gets." But she wholeheartedly defended the effort because ultimately, she said, "it tells us the answers to really important questions, like 'Where are we?' and 'Where are we going?' It contributes to assessments of costs and benefits, which can ultimately help policymakers think about where money needs to move, and it allows us to measure equity. I think we can make people's lives better by knowing what is going on in the sectors of health and health care."

10

Building Healthy Cities

KATE DESANTIS, M.ARCH, URBAN DESIGNER, GEHL INSTITUTE

GIL PENALOSA, MBA, PHDHC, CSP, FOUNDER AND CHAIR OF THE BOARD,
8 80 CITIES

ELA RAUSCH, MPP, SENIOR PROJECT MANAGER, FEDERAL RESERVE BANK
OF MINNEAPOLIS

Americans are largely an urban people. Eighty percent of the U.S. population lives in cities, defined by the Census as "densely developed residential, commercial and other nonresidential areas." Mostly, they cluster in urban settings with 50,000 or more residents.

Over the next 45 years, 100 million more people will be living on American soil, and almost all of them will be urban dwellers. To accommodate healthy living, the existing infrastructure will have to be maintained, upgraded, and expanded. Tens of millions of new housing units, along with schools, health care, and retail and commercial development, will have to be brought online. New transportation, public services, recreation, and modern communication will be needed.

What will all of that look like? Will the communities of the future accommodate walking and social engagement? Can they help promote equity or will they worsen the racial and economic divide? What should a city designed to build a Culture of Health look like?

To help answer those questions, this chapter draws on the work of these contributors.

Cities That Work For All

How do we want to live? Once we agree on how we want to live, a lot of the other decisions are going to be very easy.—Gil Penalosa

Building healthy cities begins by imagining them, said Gil Penalosa. "Just im-agine" that our children and youth can get to their activities without having to depend on someone to drive them. Imagine that older adults could age in place, as so many prefer. Imagine that the structure of daily life diminishes obesity, de-pression, and anxiety. Imagine that our communities foster a sense of belonging, improve safety, allow us to connect with nature, and give us more time to spend with friends.

The good news is that what begins as an act of imagination can actually be ac-complished. All it takes is creativity, the will to act, new mind sets, and a strategy to curb the power of what Penalosa calls the CAVE people—that is, Citizens Against Virtually Everything.

Numerous metrics tell us our cities currently lack many of the attributes that promote a Culture of Health, and that inequity is growing in some arenas. Life expectancy varies greatly across neighborhoods in the same cities, and dis-parities in the quality of schools, the availability of fresh food, and the ratio of parks to residents are well documented. A single statistic stands in for countless more: in South Fresno, California there is one acre of parkland per 1,000 resi-dents while in North Fresno, there are 4.6 acres of parks for the same number of people.

The 880 Cities initiative, launched by Penalosa, offers a powerful frame in which to make better decisions about what our cities should look like, and to change some of the indicators of inequity. The founding principle is that everything that happens in urban environments—from building parks, sidewalks, plazas, and street crossings to locating schools and hospitals – honors a commitment to make them work for someone who is eight and for someone who is 80. Think of that child and that elderly person as "in-dicator species"—when they feel confident walking across an intersection to purchase a quart of milk, we know it is safe for almost anyone to do so. Penalosa exhorts, "We've got to stop building cities as if everybody was 30 years old and athletic. Let's evaluate cities by how we treat our most vul-nerable people."

A Vibrant Commons

Sustainable mobility and thriving public places are key elements of a Culture of Health, in Penalosa's view. Investing in other-than-automobile modes of transportation is one of the great opportunities to create urban settings that put people first while benefitting health and the environment, and saving house-holds significant amounts of money. A two-car family spends an average of

20 to 30 percent of its income on mobility, and in lower-income homes that figure jumps even higher, consuming as much as one-third of family income. Conversely, with good mass transit, walking, and bicycling options in place, the costs may drop to as little as five percent of income.

Taking the steps necessary to build healthy, vibrant cities is mostly a matter of will, not money. "Citizens pay us to get things done, not to find excuses," emphasized Penalosa, describing three "doable actions" that illustrate the potential when forces are aligned to do them:

- Make parks and play available everywhere
- Open up the streets
- Make it safe to walk

Make Parks and Play Available Everywhere

For children, playing is learning—enhancing muscle strength and coordination, nurturing cognitive thinking and concentration, fostering friendships and a sense of belonging.

Investing in parks is the obvious starting strategy for creating opportunities to play. Bogota, Colombia, where Penalosa served as parks commissioner, shows what can happen when government steps in. The city built some 800 parks over five years, bringing in a mix of large parks that serve the entire city, medium-sized parks that offer room for soccer and other sports, and small neighborhood parks that encourage community and a sense of belonging. Linear parks have a special place in the mix because they can connect disparate neighborhoods, encouraging people of all economic stripes to share the same amenities.

"The whole city should be a playful city," said Penalosa, and with the right commitments, it can be. "Let's say as a goal that every child in America must have a park or a play area within a short walk, within a quarter of a mile. Everyone. But not in 40 years. In four. By 2020. It's totally doable."

If there is not a park in the neighborhood, and no easy way to develop one, planners can turn toward other shared resources. With a little creativity, play can be introduced in the schools, the sidewalks, the streets, City Hall, or the library. In New York City, a Schoolyards to Playgrounds program, created through a partnership with the Department of Education, the Department of Parks & Recreation, and the Trust for Public Land, has opened hundreds of new recreational sites for public use after school and on weekends, without the need to purchase a single acre of land.

Open Up the Streets

Streets represent 30 to 40 percent of the space in the average city. On Sundays and holidays, Bogota capitalizes on that amenity, closing the streets to cars, opening them up to people, and bringing the world's largest pop-up park to life. The city's Ciclovia initiative, which began with just a few miles of roadway in the late 1970s, expanded exponentially in the 1990s, and now stretches for 70 miles. "Magic happens," said Penalosa, as the young and the old, the rich and the poor—more than 1.5 million people every week—pour out to walk, run, bike, or skate, practice tai chi and aerobics, and sometimes to do the cha-cha. All of that with no capital investment, and without shutting down the city, because major intersections generally remain open for cars to cross.

Open streets have found champions across the United States, not only in wealthy places like Portland, Ore., and San Francisco but also in those struggling economically, like Brownsville, Texas, and San Jose, Calif. While each city takes a slightly different approach, the common theme is that the streets became a haven. And gaining health benefits doesn't require athletic prowess, only the willingness to spend time outside and join in the fun.

Another common denominator of open street programs is that people from all walks of life share the same space. That's not common in society—there is a tendency across class lines to live apart, attend separate schools, and eat at different restaurants. But when city streets are cleared of traffic, everyone from the owners of the biggest corporations to the minimum-wage workers can meet as equals. As Penalosa observes, "It doesn't matter if you have a $5,000 bike or a $50 bike. Everybody has as much fun."

Make It Safe to Walk

Walking is an almost universal human activity, the way a trip of any length begins and ends, regardless of the weather, the destination, or the additional modes of transport involved. People were built to walk, and to use all of their senses as they do. In the United States, more than one-quarter of all trips are less than a mile, and almost half are less than three miles, distances that are easy for many people to cover on foot or bicycle.

But the streets have to be safe to encourage that, and too often they are not. In the past 10 years, 47,000 pedestrians in the United States were struck and killed by drivers. In 2015 alone, 70,000 people were hit by cars as they walked. "These are not accidents, they are incidents, because most of them could have been avoided," Penalosa asserted.

Lowering traffic speed is one of the most important policy actions to improve walkability. A pedestrian struck by a car traveling 20 miles per hour stands a five percent chance of being killed; at 40 miles per hour, the probability is greater than 80 percent. For that reason, school zones typically have 20 mph speed limits. But protecting children in front of schools is not enough—promoting safety for everyone, everywhere, includes applying speed restrictions to all residential streets. Also fundamental to safety is the use of small islands on crosswalks, which could eliminate more than half of the incidents that occur at intersections.

From Talking to Doing

Penalosa identified five necessary elements for action:

- **Develop a sense of urgency.** We need to create a shared "reason why" we need to change and then do it. It can be population growth, or a public health crisis, or another shared by the specific community.
- **Generate political will** that declares "the general interest must prevail."
- **Cultivate champions.** "We need champions who will look for the solutions to the problems, not the problems for the solutions."
- **Grow leaders.** "Not one or two—we need hundreds, thousands, in the schools, in the neighborhoods, in business."
- **Engage citizens.** We learn what people really want from their parks, streets, and communities only when we listen to them.

Ultimately, Penalosa asserts that the challenges to building communities that create a Culture of Health are neither technical nor financial, but rather are political. Moving forward requires broad alliances that bring together local, state, and national elected officials; public sector workers in health, planning, parks and recreation, education, economic development, and the environment; and the community, including residents, activists, businesses, media, and faith groups. Their collective energy can transform cities and improve the quality of life of all citizens.

Public Life in the Plazas of New York

Narrowing in on one dimension of public space, Kate DeSantis described a study of how plazas promote interaction and influence social cohesion in New York City neighborhoods. Gehl, which puts architects, urban planners, cultural anthropologists, and others together to shape people-oriented cities, collaborated on the project with the J. Max Bond Center on Design for the Just City.

The team studied seven of the more than 70 plazas created under New York City's Plaza Program, which together have transformed 400,000 square feet of underused streets and awkward intersections into public space since 2010. Built quickly and on low budgets, these plazas usually have moveable street furniture and planters that can be altered based on experience. The plazas require local initiative to launch so end users have "skin in the game." Communities apply for funding from the Department of Transportation, and are then required to maintain and manage the space in keeping with city guidelines.

Two of the plazas studied are in Manhattan and five are in the outer boroughs—two in Queens and three in Brooklyn. The Manhattan plazas are adjacent to commercial and mixed-use buildings, and tend to attract a more transient population, compared to the outer-borough plazas, which mostly draw local people from surrounding residential neighborhoods.

Although conventional techniques for assessing return-on-investment from public spaces (for example, through increased retail sales and fewer storefront vacancies) are available, research designs to measure how the space supports better health outcomes are less well established. This study used a mixed-method approach that included:

- Desktop research provided baseline Census-tract information within a half-mile of each plaza.
- Observational studies, which documented what happens on the ground. For 12-hour periods, on both weekdays and weekends, trained volunteers recorded the nature and level of daily activity—noting whether people were sitting or standing, doing yoga or playing, walking through without stopping, waiting for the bus—and the time of day they were likely to do it.
- Intercept surveys of almost 500 people offered insights about how they felt about the space.
- Interviews with plaza managers highlighted any management constraints or financial concerns.

These methods reveal what actually happens in the plaza, rather than what people might claim at a meeting that they want. "We call it voting with your feet," said DeSantis. "People don't necessarily plan to go do something, but they found themselves in this space and met someone new and now they want to come back."

Among finding highlights:

- Sixty-seven percent of people surveyed said that plazas in their local communities had increased the time they spend outside. That figure was even higher where nearby public space was in short supply (such as in Corona, Queens, where almost 80 percent of respondents were spending more time outdoors as a result of the plaza).

- Almost two-thirds of the people using the plazas had walked to them, indicating that they lived or worked nearby, and were either passing through or taking a pause from other activities.
- Users of the smaller outer-borough plazas reported a strong sense of ownership. Although only three percent had been involved in planning the plaza, more than 75 percent answered "yes" when asked, "Is this your plaza?" That rate was significantly lower in Manhattan, where the population tends to be less local.
- Fifty-three percent of users across all seven plazas said they recognized more people, or had met someone new. That percent was higher in the outerborough plazas and among people earning less than $50,000/year.
- Lower-income groups are overrepresented in the plazas, compared to the surrounding neighborhoods. For example, 49 percent of the people who actually use the plazas surrounding Manhattan's Meatpacking Plaza had incomes below $50,000, compared to 26 percent of those who live in the neighborhood.

Associating very specific health outcomes with new public space is difficult, given differences in the size and configuration of the plazas, and in the sociodemographic makeup of the surrounding community. But as data accumulate and the plaza program continues to expand in New York, they hint at "city-making approaches" that can infuse a neighborhood with new vitality. By introducing the kinds of swift changes described here, and then measuring what happens as rigorously as possible, a feedback loop is created that can inform design changes. And that, in turn, invites more people in. DeSantis concludes, "We can increase physical activity and increase social capital in our communities by making local space that people feel they have a sense of ownership over."

Community Development and Health

One of the most promising new partners in community development is the health care sector.—Ben Bernanke, Federal Reserve Board of Governors

Another lens on the built environment emerges from the Federal Reserve Community Development function. The Bank's Community Development Department's role is to foster economic opportunity in low- to moderate-income communities. In recent years, their economic development efforts have expanded to include health and early childhood development. In 2010, RWJF reached out to the Federal Reserve System asking for help in exploring influences on health that fall outside the health care system. Since then, the Fed has held more than 20 meetings that brought community development and health practitioners together to learn more about each other's work, and has expanded its activities in this arena since then.

Community development efforts contribute to all four of the Action Areas that undergird the Culture of Health Framework, observed Ela Rausch. The connection to creating healthy communities is perhaps most apparent, but the process also involves gathering input from local residents, presenting opportunities to make health a shared value; fostering cross-sector collaborations; and integrating health services and systems by encouraging hospitals to reach beyond their institutional walls and expand on their anchor mission.

Examples of how community development and health are working together to enhance the built environment can be seen in many venues—hospitals partnering with Community Development Financial Institutions (CDFIs) to build affordable housing; farmer's markets located in hospitals; county public health departments supporting small business owners; and federally qualified health centers teaming up with grocery stores. "The built environment presents a common playing field for different departments—county public health and county parks and recreation; city public health and city public works—to come together and share resources" said Rausch.

But barriers still arise frequently, and answers to difficult questions are needed to overcome them:

- **High development costs:** How do we reduce barriers to investment in low- and moderate-income communities?
- **Zoning and regulation:** How can we change policies, or create new ones, that promote opportunities for building, instead of restricting them, as has been the historic pattern?
- **Lack of site control:** Who owns the land, who makes decisions about its use, and can we transfer control to those in a better position to make decisions that benefit the community?
- **Lack of infrastructure:** Are there development solutions that don't require a significant investment in infrastructure (such as mobile food markets)?
- **Low population density:** How do we meet transportation and other needs in areas that lack urban density?
- **NIMBYism:** How do we change attitudes and gather the political will to move past the not-in-my-backyard syndrome?
- **Lack of shared knowledge and collaboration:** How do we measure the impact of community development projects that influence health?

With support from RWJF, the Federal Reserve Bank of Minneapolis and Wilder Research developed the Metrics for Healthy Communities website (see *www.metricsforhealthycommunities.org*), which offers a tool for evaluating community health improvement initiatives. "One of the things that we kept hearing over and over from community development and health practitioners was that lack of access to shared data and shared measures made collaboration difficult," Rausch said.

To inform the research that led to the development of the site, the Federal Reserve Bank of Minneapolis conducted a national survey of more than 600 community development and health professionals, asking: "What do you measure? How do you measure? What data sources do you use? Do you have any good advice for measurement?"

Ultimately, researchers compiled more than 180 measures and organized them into six logic models representing aspects of the built environment that are especially rich in cross-sector opportunities to improve health—affordable housing, child-care centers, community health centers, access to fresh produce, physical activity, and supportive housing. These logic models incorporate as many of the RWJF Action Framework elements as possible.

Each logic model briefly describes a topic's influence on the social determinants of health, and offers a menu of activities to help achieve identified goals. The menu also suggests measurable short-, medium-, and long-term outcomes; provides links to available data sources, from the local to the national scale; describes methods for collecting original data; and offers other advice to drive effective cross-sector partnerships that include both community development and health actors.

Reflections on Building for Health

As the initiatives described here illustrate, public health has an active role to play in shaping a built environment that supports and celebrates well-being. Rausch urged people in the field to "inject yourself into the conversation." Added Penalosa, "Become champions."

The theme of partnership echoed repeatedly across the discussion. Too often, the failure to build bridges impedes powerful "city-making," said DeSantis. "If we can find a more common vision under which to make and shape cities, our policy could better align with our transportation initiatives, could better align with how we develop buildings, could better align with our open space initiatives. They all tend to be separate and managed by different groups and different people with different expertise."

But Penalosa pointed out that it may be possible to exploit those differences in pursuit of a single vision. One official may be indifferent to parks but deeply concerned about public health, while another may see the environment or economic development as top priorities. From their many angles, each can recognize the advantage of investing in recreation, so identifying the resonant arguments for each decision-maker can help everyone drive toward the same endpoint.

The "green building" movement, which helped integrate sustainability into the real estate industry, suggests advocacy strategies that might also contribute to the movement for healthy places. One element is understanding what motivates individuals who have authority to act. "Every person in the chain of decision-making in the built environment has a client or needs a mandate of some type," said audience member Matt Trowbridge, MPH, MD, associate professor at the University of Virginia School of Medicine. "What does a mayor need, what does an architect need, what does somebody at the Federal Reserve need to take action towards promoting healthy places in each of those roles?"

DeSantis underscored the value of measurement as a compass showing where we need to head. The premise, she said, is that "you should measure what you care about. Let's test an idea and then measure it and understand as best we can what the data says, and then change what we do—that is a way of working we need to do more."

Penalosa seconded the need for action-oriented research. "A study doesn't get finished when it gets published in a journal. It gets finished when the findings are implemented. I think we need to move away from doing interesting studies to doing useful studies."

Audience member John Moon, MPP, district manager of community development for the Federal Reserve Bank of San Francisco, called for more local participation in decisions that alter the built environment. The disparities in the built environment did not occur by accident, but rather were the result of market forces, political forces and planning decisions, he said. Reversing their influence requires "getting to the issue of community voice and empowerment. It's really important to tap into, and lift up, communities so they are able to contribute, and have the technical know-how to respond to a consolidated plan or to mobilize."

Ultimately, improving the built environment—whether through biking and walking paths, public transportation, recreational facilities, affordable housing, or lively public spaces—is a means, not an end in itself. The real goal of a successful city is to distribute resources equitably so that inhabitants can live healthier and happier lives. As DeSantis puts it, "We need to start thinking of the built environment as the tool to get to the outcomes we want to achieve."

Gathering the data that document the influence of the built environment on health, and then using the data to guide action, are key steps forward.

11

Rethinking How We Police Communities

AMANDA GELLER, PHD, CLINICAL ASSOCIATE PROFESSOR
OF SOCIOLOGY, NEW YORK UNIVERSITY

JOHN RICH, MD, MPH, PROFESSOR, DORNSIFE SCHOOL OF PUBLIC
HEALTH AT DREXEL UNIVERSITY, AND AUTHOR OF *WRONG PLACE,
WRONG TIME: TRAUMA AND VIOLENCE IN THE LIVES
OF YOUNG BLACK MEN*

AUKE VAN DIJK, ADVISOR TO THE POLICE CHIEF IN AMSTERDAM,
THE NETHERLANDS, AND STRATEGIST, AGORA POLICE & SECURITY

We are using policing to solve way too many problems that are not going to be solved by violent imposition of control.—Scott Burris, JD

Over the past several years, the clashes between police and the people they are sworn to protect have been a too common news story. Eric Garner, Freddie Gray, and Michael Brown became household symbols of stop-and-frisk tactics, police have faced intense legal scrutiny, and a groundswell of rage swept through Ferguson, Missouri; Baltimore, Maryland; St. Paul, Minnesota; and other American cities.

Among people living in the communities of color where frequent police encounters are the norm, the defects in the system have been increasingly revealed to have significant health consequences. Indeed, said panel moderator Scott Burris, JD, Professor of Law at Temple Law School, "the level of misery that the status quo visits on a large portion of the population" is nowhere more acute than in the interactions between policing and the policed.

The dysfunctional relationship also takes its victims among law enforcers. In Dallas, a sniper ambushed and killed five officers during a peaceful protest against fatal police shootings. High rates of suicide within the policing profession reveal anguish at its most intense.

Neither the health care nor the criminal justice systems have been particularly successful at addressing the trauma associated with policing gone wrong. Both fields spend much of their time "reacting and treating acute bad things that are happening in our communities," said Burris, but the social and economic structures and pathologies at their root have often been beyond reach.

Public health offers a different set of tools for repairing the harms that are occurring daily in American communities. An important theme of this panel was how the field can take a leadership role that will help engage policing as an ally in building a Culture of Health.

At the Intersection of Public Health and Policing

Law enforcement and public health are fundamentally related and share objectives and ways of working, although they are characterized by a different culture and language.—Auke van Dijk

Auke van Dijk mapped out the territory that connects law enforcement and public health. At the most abstract level, he said, the fields share the core value of freedom—it is the province of both public health and law enforcement to protect the population from the fear of ill health, injury, and deaths that are unnatural and untimely.

More specifically, van Dijk cited substance use, violence prevention, mental health, sexual exploitation of children, public disorder, emergency response, trauma, and bioterrorism as examples of shared concerns. As well, engaging with vulnerable groups and marginalized communities is an essential component of each agenda.

Policing and public health both involve numerous stakeholders and target their interventions in many contexts across the physical environment, the social environment, and the individual. There are similarities, too, in the continuum of interventions available to them, which run from a participatory, community-based approach focused on prevention to authoritarian enforcement of regulations and laws. No single strategy can be assumed to be superior, emphasized van Dijk; indeed, any combination can be justified, depending on circumstances.

Opportunities for policing and public health to work together likewise lie on a continuum. Some tasks are of necessity performed completely in isolation from each other while others work best with a fully integrated team. The degree of engagement depends on, and will influence, how knowledge is used, interventions are designed, and policies are integrated. Again, no one approach will be appropriate in every situation.

Given the many common threads, what gets in the way of promising initiatives to move the fields toward each other? The simple answer, said van Dijk, is that this is a new area, at the edges of well-established policies, structures, and disciplines. By definition, many players with various mandates, goals, and norms are involved, and bringing them together requires that alternative institutional arrangements be designed. Existing organizational, cultural, and intellectual siloes lend complexity to that effort.

All of that speaks to the imperative of growing leaders who can operate where law enforcement and public health intersect. Leadership in this "emergent domain," as van Dijk characterizes it, will look fundamentally different from leadership focused primarily on the aims of a single organization.

In both arenas, community engagement is a key strategy for translating intention into meaningful action. Public health has over the past few decades become infused with ideas about empowerment, social capital, and the importance of seeing individuals within the context of their communities. "This evolution," said van Dijk, "is matched by the philosophy of community policing, which reflects many of the same influences and approaches."

With the legitimacy of police under pressure, not only in the United States but elsewhere in the world, signing on to a health agenda may be crucial to the policing of the future. According to van Dijk, "Increasingly, holistic models of community safety and well-being are at the core of strategy development in both law enforcement and public health." What van Dijk referred to as the "policing web" of prevention, deterrence, and enforcement recognizes crime as a subset of harm and takes responsibility for risk in ways that go well beyond the traditional domains of policing.

The Health Consequences of Stop-and-Frisk

> *We generally find a link between what people experience in their own personal encounters with their perceptions of the institution as a whole. We think that the diminished legitimacy of the police could have implications for the community more broadly.*—Amanda Geller

If van Dijk's presentation laid out a hopeful vision for an approach to 21st-century policing that is better aligned with public health considerations, the realities on the ground show how far it is from being fully realized. Research has long revealed mass incarceration and many other features of the criminal justice system to be significant drivers of adverse health outcomes, but more recently, the health impacts of less severe encounters with the police have also gained attention. Amanda Geller's presentation explored the risks and consequences.

Despite dramatic declines in rates of serious crime since the 1980s, a philosophy of "proactive policing" has significantly increased the exposure of urban residents to the police. Geller cautioned that this is not an inevitably antagonistic event. Although a narrow enforcement model is often applied, community-involved styles of policing are also the coinage in many settings. But the encounter does frequently spark conflict, and the widespread use of stop-and-frisk activity—"Terry stops" in the legal lexicon—has certainly been a factor.

Over a 10-year period, the New York City Police Department initiated more than 4.4 million stop-and-frisk encounters, the vast majority (88 percent) young men of color. At their peak in 2011, more than 700,000 stops occurred, giving New York the dubious distinction of being a national leader in this arena. Most individuals stopped had done nothing wrong—only about 6 percent of stops led to an arrest, and another 6 percent resulted in a summons of some sort.

Stop-and-frisk experiences are often aggressive, with half of them involving some form of physical contact with the police. Some are edged with racial invectives and taunts about an individual's masculinity. An emerging literature suggests there are health implications to that kind of behavior in the form of psychological trauma and physical manifestations of stress.

Geller sought to learn more about those and other outcomes by surveying 1,200 young men by telephone, with systematic oversampling in high-stop neighborhoods. Measures included symptoms of anxiety and post-traumatic stress disorder (PTSD) and examined both internalized stigma and perceptions of structural stigma associated with the police. They also asked subjects whether they thought the stop had been conducted fairly, whether the officer respected their rights, and whether they believed the outcome was what they deserved under the law.

Key findings from the study:

• Young men who reported more intrusive stops over the previous year also reported more symptoms of anxiety and PTSD.
• Symptom levels were most elevated at the far end of the intrusion distribution—that is, the 5 to 10 percent of men who reported the most invasive stops showed the strongest association between the experience and health outcomes.
• There was some moderation of symptoms among men who felt they had received procedural justice during their stops, although this finding was inconsistent.

- Men who reported more intrusive stops had diminished perceptions of the legitimacy of the police, and were less willing to cooperate with the law.
- Men who perceived their encounters as legally conducted had more positive perceptions of police legitimacy.
- Perceptions of procedural justice and police legitimacy were associated with broader measures of civic participation, and predicted such behaviors as obeying the law, cooperating with police investigations, and willingness to serve on a jury.

Geller highlighted some limitations in the findings. For one, the direction of the causal relationship cannot be assumed, especially if police are more likely to stop individuals who display mental health symptoms or if those symptoms are more likely to escalate a situation. As well, it is possible that individuals willing to talk at length about their experiences have had particularly unsettling encounters.

But the correlations are nonetheless cause for concern. New York City's former Police Commissioner Raymond Kelly has asserted that stop-and-frisk is simply a fact of urban life that residents should accept, implying that its consequences are minor. Geller's findings indicate otherwise.

Trauma and the Cycle of Violence

John Rich used the power of narrative to sketch a world inhabited by many young men of color, for whom random violence is a regular occurrence and contact with the police is routine. Part of his message was that in communities steeped in racism and brutality, the police are far from the only traumatizing force. Rather, many types of trauma build upon one another, cumulatively influencing the ways in which young people see the many systems that surround them.

As damaging as that reality is, it also contains the kernel of a solution—the possibility of aligning systems to heal, rather than harm. Healing Hurt People, a community-focused, hospital-based program in Philadelphia, takes aims at trauma with a well-coordinated package designed to interrupt the cycle of violence and improve overall health. As part of that initiative, young people attend a week-long workshop in which they produce a digital story about their own lives, as they wish them to be told.

Rich introduced one participant, a young man who was shooting baskets the first time he watched someone get shot and later lost his cousin and brother to guns. In the aftermath of that terror, the man described nightmares, loneliness, awakening in tears, and a foreboding certainty that he, too, would take a bullet. In a vivid display of post-traumatic stress, he began to angle his body as he walked down the street, hoping the bullet would hit only his shoulder, and not his heart. "None of the people I knew in the sandbox is alive today," he confided.

But even as he found himself "looking back over my shoulder, in my own shadow," this young man also spoke of hope, a yearning "that one day I will stop focusing on my past and start looking ahead to my future." Who could argue against the wisdom of supporting that aspiration?

The lingering emotions of a violent encounter are often linked not only to the incident itself, but to its follow-up, as Rich made vivid with the story of a man named Jimmy, who was shot six times in an act of revenge. As he was loaded onto a stretcher, carried down two flights of stairs, and placed in an ambulance, an officer on the scene peppered him with the same question over and over: "Who shot you? Who shot you?"

Jimmy kept saying he didn't know, but the officer persisted, escalating the tension with a somber declaration: "Jimmy, you got shot six times, man. You ain't going to make it. You're going to die. Who shot you? Who shot you?"

As he lay bleeding, Jimmy recalled his assumption that the cop must be right: "So I'm thinking I'm not going to make it either."

Again came the push. "Come on, man, you ain't going to make it. Who shot you?"

"I'm like, 'Man, I do not know who shot me. I'm sitting up here bleedin' to death. Could you all take me to the hospital, please?' "

Rich urged his audience to consider what might happen when Jimmy finally arrives at the emergency department, where no knows what transpired, and is likely to see only a panicked or uncooperative young man. It is hard not to conclude, as Rich does, that "this tactic, traumatic as it is in this case ineffective, informs the way in which this young person will see this experience down the road."

One man's fear and another's sense of duty is revealed in that clash of interests. Where is the training, and the wisdom, that would have allowed officers to handle the situation differently?

Another kind of encounter, captured on a video that later went viral, could also produce enduring damage. There, a man holding a baby girl reportedly jumped over a turnstile at a Philadelphia subway station. Moments later, an officer approached him on the train and, after several minutes of discussion, appeared to grab the passenger by the throat. The altercation ended with the man handcuffed and led back onto the platform, still clutching his daughter. In a subsequent investigation, the officer told the police chief that he thought he would have been disciplined had he not acted on an apparent fare evasion.

"Yet there was a child in the midst of this," Rich emphasized. "In terms of system alignment, what if everybody was aligned toward the well-being of the child? Would the police officer, the system, have been aligned to make this not a big issue?" A local resident lamented, "They're supposed to help us, they're supposed to protect us, we supposed to look for them to help, but they the ones, you know, that's helping destroy. That's the crazy part."

As with stop-and-frisk incidents, such interactions cause local residents to question the priorities of the police. Even if they are not violent themselves, they can spark a cycle of violence. "If you don't believe that the police will protect you and you're hyperaroused, then weapons become a logical alternative for self-protection," said Rich.

Reflections on Research

The imperative of taming the relationship between policing and community and rebuilding security as a core element of health is evident in both data and story. But further research is crucial to document the nature, extent, and cause of the challenges, and to provide actionable intelligence about the best ways to redirect resources. Tested models remain in short supply.

Recognizing the urgent need for healing, John Rich called for the pairing of learning with action as a research agenda is developed. He described design thinking that distinguishes "looking" (which researchers might think of as gathering data), "understanding" (data analysis), and ultimately the more action-oriented "making." "Can we forge research that allows our learning to be iterative and embeds the studying within the doing?" he asked.

Rich also underscored the importance of bringing voices from the community into the work, especially those of young people. Creating opportunities for them to tell their stories, and to participate as co-researchers, helps narrow the lens to issues that are most salient in particular settings. While some measures and strategies may appropriately apply to many contexts, vigorous local engagement will surely identify others that are unique.

Among avenues for future research:

System change: What practical rules and design principles will provide a framework for systems change that brings public health and policing closer? Evidence should support conclusions that are relevant to operations in a specific time and place, rather than prescriptive statements that ignore temporal and geographic context. "It is really important to focus on the relationships between mechanisms, contexts, and outcomes," urged van Dijk.

Health outcomes: What is the influence of police encounters on health over time? Given hints that even minimal encounters may induce trauma, transparent and detailed data from both health care providers and the police will allow for a more nuanced understanding of these interrelationships.

A "life course" perspective on young people: How does prior trauma drive subsequent responses? Research focused on the journey that young people have taken through health care, criminal justice, schools, and other institutions can help explain how interactions between individuals and systems can become flashpoints, and how to avoid kindling that fire.

Measuring exposure and impact: What measures allow clinicians to screen for exposure to trauma? How are the extent and intensity of continued stress and PTSD best gauged? Just as clinicians routinely screen for lead exposure and mental health problems, they might also ask about interactions with the police. Collecting these kinds of data, and then sharing them with the community, can inform policy and practice.

Preparation for injustice: How does the assumption of negative experiences—the young man anticipating a shooting, the parent educating his black son about how to stay safe when questioned by the police—enter into the calculation of stress? The foundation of trust is shaky indeed when children in communities of color are warned not to run while they are outside, or to keep their hands out of their pockets while shopping, lest they be accused of shoplifting.

Trauma in the lives of police: How much do we know about the trauma that police officers have experienced, and how does it influence their behavior? Empirical research may reveal links between a history of adversity and how they interpret and respond to threats.

From strategic vision to operational action: What needs to happen to ensure that police on the front lines have the competencies, knowledge, skills, and attitudes to implement strategies that have been tested and found to be sound? Training is needed to translate high-level thinking about organizational culture and direction into language that resonates with the officers who interact daily with populations that have complex social and health needs. A crucial component of this is the development of a collaborative world-view.

Reflections on Policy and Practice

Policing is at a perilous turning point and its future remains opaque and uncertain. Policing is reinventing itself, so please seize the moment.
—Auke van Dijk

If any measure of solace can be taken from the clashes between police and the community that have jolted the nation, it is that they have forced more attention on the importance of collaboration across sectors to revisit and rethink the fundamental implications of police and community relations. Policymakers and practitioners in both the legal and public health arenas are deepening their conversations about system failures and opportunities amidst a call to look beyond individual incidents to root causes.

The current dialogue builds on the recognition that policing is critical to community well-being and not inherently repressive. Communities need the police, none more so than those who are most likely to be the victims of violence. But policing by consent is the more effective and sustainable model, more conducive to generating health than policing by control, said van Dijk. He called the effectiveness of a narrow view of law enforcement built largely on arrests and imprisonment "near zero."

Unsurprisingly, themes of police legitimacy and systems alignment infused the panel discussions. Geller's stop-and-frisk findings reinforced the conclusions of Tom Tyler's seminal work of legal scholarship, which argued, essentially, that police need public support and cooperation to be effective, and that such support only comes when people believe the police are exercising their authority appropriately.

All too often, that is not the case. Instead, a "baseline expectation of being treated unfairly by the police" is being met, warns Rich. By way of example, he contrasted norms in two settings. The default in the suburbs is likely to be taking home a child who has been drinking, or otherwise gotten himself into trouble. In urban environments, "where there is a much dimmer view of the community and family, there's not even an idea that you can take this child home," he said. That kind of disparity builds dangerous synergy, with the assumptions of the police about the community matched by community assumptions about the police.

While core policing will always require a degree of split-second decision-making, said Geller, officers also need to deepen their understanding of the neighborhoods they serve, and develop the skills to engage appropriately with people who have been traumatized. The imperative of stronger ties within the community is also made vivid by the challenges that can ensue when police and health care providers meet for the first time in a hospital emergency department, each bringing with them very different concerns about the victim.

Collaboration with other community-serving organizations is one way to begin aligning systems. In the Netherlands, for example, police officers and psychiatric nurses often work together on the front lines. Joe Marx, adviser and senior communications officer at the Robert Wood Johnson Foundation, described a "lightbulb moment" when health system leaders and law enforcement leaders in Spartanburg, S.C., sat down together to look at data about those in the community that were the most frequent users of emergency health services. They discovered they were serving many of the same people—but the clinicians saw them as patients and the police knew them as prisoners. It was an example of silo-busting, as advocated in an earlier chapter in this book, *The Secrecy Divide: Sharing Data Across Sectors*, and the result was a decision to introduce mental health and substance abuse counseling into the prison system with an eye toward providing upstream support. That change was among the prevention approaches that helped the community save more than $40 million in health care costs in just five years.

A history of PTSD is not only a reality in communities of color, but also a characteristic of police work as well. "A persistent specter of violence, violent incidents, and a state of continual stress can desensitize police to the way they look at the world. And what might be the potential effect of this 'steady' state of uncertainty and peril? Becoming inured and yet hypersensitive to encounters that can cause police to react quickly and instinctively when confronted with what they feel as threat, whether imagined or real," observed Dennis Andrulis, PhD, MPH, senior research scientist at the Texas Health Institute. These circumstances and their consequences, Andrulis suggested, represent a common reality with communities of color, offering an important bridge of shared experiences for communicating and understanding between two very different cultures.

Discussions among the panelists and the audience surfaced a mix of strategies within the purview of policing to lift up its role as a contributor of health. Among them:

- Police training that puts more emphasis on implicit biases and social context
- Training that teaches officers how to approach someone exhibiting PTSD
- Assessing officers themselves for PTSD and acting on red flags
- Redefining core competencies for police hires
- Integrating professionals with complementary skills into the front lines of policing

But the collective power of added skill sets, stricter accountability, and new partnerships is only part of the solution. Beyond reforms at the level of the police force lies the transdisciplinary work that can move the field from scattered "ah-ha moments" to broader system changes.

"How do we create governance strategies by which power is truly shared between health and public safety?" asked Hillary Kunins, MD, MPH, assistant commissioner at the New York City Department of Health and Mental Hygiene. Case examples of such power-sharing approaches would be useful in promoting alignment, she said.

Gary Slutkin, MD, an epidemiologist at the University of Illinois at Chicago School of Public Health, and founder of Cure Violence, went further, arguing that criminal justice is fundamentally the wrong venue for addressing violent behavior. Like smoking or risky sexual behavior, he urged that violence be viewed as a health behavior, with the health system "completely activated" to work on this problem as we do for other epidemics: "Behaviors are contagious and peer driven and in most countries are not thought to be managed by punishment anymore. It's medieval thinking and practice. It's time for the health sector to step up."

The antagonism between communities of color and the police is not a new story. It is, however, an unacceptable one that must change.

New models are clearly needed to establish bonds of trust. A first step is to define the respective contributions that the police, the health professions, and the community can make toward building a Culture of Health by working together.

Ultimately, effective partnerships require deep discussion of the nature and extent of the security a healthy society requires. Just what do we expect from policing? And, what do police expect from the communities they serve? Developing measures that can signal positive outcomes compared to the current situation can help bring law enforcement and community members together as partners in systems improvement.

Climate Change Through
a Health Lens

ERIC KLINENBERG, PHD, PROFESSOR OF SOCIOLOGY AND DIRECTOR,
INSTITUTE FOR PUBLIC KNOWLEDGE, NEW YORK UNIVERSITY,
AND RESEARCH DIRECTOR, REBUILD BY DESIGN

SABRINA MCCORMICK, PHD, SOCIOLOGIST, ASSISTANT PROFESSOR,
GEORGE WASHING UNIVERSITY, ASSOCIATE PRODUCER,
THE YEARS OF LIVING DANGEROUSLY

LINDA RUDOLPH, MD, MPH, DIRECTOR, PUBLIC HEALTH INSTITUTE'S
CENTER FOR CLIMATE CHANGE AND HEALTH, AND FORMER DEPUTY
DIRECTOR, CALIFORNIA DEPARTMENT OF PUBLIC HEALTH'S CENTER
FOR CHRONIC DISEASE PREVENTION AND HEALTH

These kinds of conversations are the beginning of something that we will be working on the rest of our lives.—Eric Klinenberg

Climate change is often identified as an environmental issue, but it also has very real health consequences that have a disproportionate impact on disadvantaged populations in the United States and globally.

The Culture of Health lens embraces the comprehensive climate and health assessment by the U.S. Global Change Research Program, which has concluded that climate change related to extreme heat, severe storms, flooding, droughts, compromised air quality, a rise in vector-borne disease, and sea-level changes is a growing threat to human health and well-being: "Climate and health impacts do not occur in isolation, and an individual or community could face multiple threats at the same time, at different stages in one's life, or accumulating over the course of one's life."

Extreme heat, for example, can "exacerbate asthma, trigger heart attacks and strokes, and lead to death," wrote Alonzo L. Plough, PhD, MPH, vice president,

Research-Evaluation-Learning and chief science officer at RWJF. "Droughts affect food production and prices, and can contribute to increased malnutrition and undernutrition. Those who are already vulnerable—who live in communities where it's not uncommon for standing water to create a breeding ground for vector-borne diseases after heavy storms; where air quality is bad; and where buildings tend to be older and poorly maintained—also stand to be most affected by climate change."

From their diverse backgrounds in public health, sociology, documentary filmmaking, and the study of the built environment, the contributors presented specific examples of the health threats posed by climate change; emphasized intergenerational equity, given that decisions made today will influence the health of generations to come; noted optimistically that actions to reverse or lessen climate changes actually present remarkable health opportunities; and promoted a sense of urgency at a time when some still question the reality of climate change.

The Health Impacts of Climate Change

Every aspect of climate change impacts health in multiple ways. And in almost every one of those ways there's disproportionate impacts on people of color, low-income people in already disadvantaged communities, and people with chronic illness—whether you look at that within the United States or globally.—Linda Rudolph

Why is climate change a *health* issue? Linda Rudolph not only asked this question but she answered it, calling the health impacts of climate change "profound, complex, and diverse."

The growing list of climate change consequences follows different pathways, "but all end up impacting health," said Rudolph, the principal investigator on a Public Health Institute project to advance the integration of health into the policies of local jurisdictions around California. Consider:

• **Direct impacts of extreme heat and extreme weather:** In this category, Rudolph listed illnesses and death associated with high temperatures; injuries and deaths from storms and floods; and damages to housing and crops, and the accompanying displacement and food supply shortages.

Rudolph pointed out that the United States has already experienced climate changes as a threat to the food and water supply, particularly in areas where it has reduced snow packs and exacerbated drought. She noted that in California, "we've got thousands of households that literally don't have tap water anymore because their wells have run dry."

- **Indirect impacts of global warming:** Here, Rudolph specifically cited rising ozone levels, which "exacerbate our existing air pollution problems" and impact crop yields. Drought and water-related disasters add further havoc to crop yields, which in turn increases food costs and drives food insecurity. More unexpectedly, policy responses to climate change can sometimes have negative consequences. For instance, increased use of corn-based ethanol for fuel made corn prices spike and had "a very significant impact on food insecurity in Mexico several years ago," Rudolph said.

   Food and water scarcities also lead to civil unrest and conflicts over land and water, and drive migration from areas where people can no longer grow food. "Many experts think that a very severe drought in Syria was a precipitating factor in the Syrian Civil War," said Rudolph.

   Rising temperatures and changing precipitation patterns also change the distribution of vector-borne diseases and patterns of pollen, which is being linked to allergies. Ocean acidification brings another package of problems, damaging fish supplies and fisheries "as a result of the ocean serving as a sink for carbon dioxide," said Rudolph. (She acknowledged that overfishing and other factors also have an impact.)

Rudolph continued to give examples of how climate change operates in multiple and sometimes unexpected ways to create a negative impact on the food supply. For example, global warming is known to increase the rate of growth of pests and weeds, which, in turn, "impels farmers to use more pesticides and herbicides with all of their attendant health impacts, particularly for farm workers."

Four lesser-known consequences of climate warming on the food chain:

- **Decreased milk production of dairy cattle.** Rudolph said a recent California drought had pushed up the price of hay, and forced grass-challenged ranchers to cull thousands of livestock because they didn't have enough to feed them.
- **Increased damage to grain supplies being transported in the global food supply chain.** For example, during the 2011-12 drought in the Midwest, large ships carrying grain to the rest of the country were backed up in ports along the Mississippi River because the river was too low in some areas for the ships to pass. Consequently, the grain shipments became moldy, rotted, and could not be used.
- **Disruption of the wine industry.** Wine growers in regions that have experienced heat waves and prolonged drought can no longer grow certain grapes, which require consistent temperatures and water levels.
- **Depressed nutritional values in food and increased outbreaks of *E. coli*.** Rising temperatures increase the risks of food-borne and water-borne illnesses, including salmonella or *E. coli* poisoning. And increased levels of

carbon dioxide in the air can "actually reduce the nutrient levels in staple crops, which is particularly important in lesser-developed nations where people are totally reliant on those staple crops to get iron, zinc, protein, and so on," Rudolph said. In her honest assessment, "the complexity of climate change and its impacts on food supply and its nutritional value is concerning, to say the least. Because we do need food and water for our basic survival."

Climate Change and Impact on Diseases

Climate change is the biggest crisis humanity has ever faced. This is not a crisis of tomorrow. It's a crisis of today.—Sabrina McCormick

When it comes to climate change and its impact on diseases, sociologist and filmmaker Sabrina McCormick did not mince words. Looking out over an audience of health care providers, scientific experts, and policymakers, she said unequivocally that "every population we work with will be affected by climate change, if they have not already been affected." The situation is dire, she added. A sense of urgency is required to address the sheer breadth and depth of its ramifications, "both in terms of mitigating and reducing greenhouse gasses as well as adapting to what we've already begun as a global crisis."

Zeroing in on vector-borne diseases, McCormick pointed specifically to the Zika and the Chikungunya viruses, both spread by mosquitoes to humans with increasing frequency as global temperatures rise. While the Chikungunya virus primarily causes joint pain, fever, and muscle aches for a week or two,[1] the Zika virus is associated with a devastating neurological birth defect called microcephaly in children whose mothers were bitten by an infected mosquito while pregnant or before becoming pregnant.[2] Paul Tarini, senior program officer at RWJF and panel moderator, referred to Zika as "the poster child for the health impacts of climate change."

"Mosquitoes, their viral load and geographic reach, are directly related to temperature. And 2015 was the hottest year on record, the hottest year mankind has ever known," noted McCormick, who is also associate professor, school of public health at George Washington University and an alumna of the RWJF Health and Society Scholars program. "This is affecting diseases like Zika, and Chikungunya, too, that are in turn causing incredible public health crises, not just in Brazil but here in the United States. We have public health emergencies around heat waves, and around other emergent diseases. It's something that our

---

[1] For more about Chikungunya virus, see *www.cdc.gov/chikungunya/symptoms/*.
[2] For more about Zika virus, see *www.cdc.gov/zika/pregnancy/index.html*.

public health systems have to be prepared for and we, as individuals, have to become educated about."

McCormick also described another rapidly growing disease tied to climate change: Valley Fever, a mold-borne disease that people acquire by breathing in the microscopic fungal spores that typically live in the ground.[3] Valley Fever is endemic to the southwestern United States and certain parts of Latin America where mold spores get kicked up in the air, which happens more frequently during periods of drought. McCormick describes how prison populations in the Southwest are especially susceptible to contracting Valley Fever, with prisons in southern California reporting rates of infection that are "up to 300 times that of the broader population." According to recent research, black men are at significantly higher risk than white men when it comes to contracting the disease, along with Filipinos and Pacific Islanders. In California, a disproportionately large number of black and brown inmates are housed in prisons in the dusty, endemic Central Valley area of the state where the disease thrives and where 16 of the state's 33 adult prisons are located.

"Valley Fever is directly connected to climate change and to the increase in drought that we see in the Southwest," she explained, noting that the disease has reportedly moved up the western seaboard into Oregon and Washington. "It's a lesser-known disease that's having incredible effects on populations that are very disadvantaged."

Impacts of Climate Change on the Built Environment

> *Climate change has become a conversation changer. It's changed the facts on the ground for people who are concerned about human welfare, well-being, settlement patterns, and vital infrastructures. When I teach students about this, I say it doesn't really matter what field you go into—this is an issue that is going to be relevant for you.* —Eric Klinenberg

Sociologist and author Eric Klinenberg began his remarks with a personal admission: "I've increasingly come to see climate change as the big context for so much of what we do. It is a tough conversation to have, but one I think that is vital."

Klinenberg has studied cities and climate change since the 1990s, when he conducted research for his first book, *Heat Wave: A Social Autopsy of Disaster in Chicago*. A recipient of RWJF's 2005 Investigator Award in Healthy Policy

---

[3] For more about Valley Fever, see *www.cdc.gov/features/valleyfever/*.

Research, his professional involvement with climate change increased significantly in 2012, following Hurricane Sandy. In 2013, he authored "Adaptation: Can
Cities be Climate-Proofed?" in *The New Yorker*, and organized a series of public
events to explore the post-Sandy context, climate change, and New York City's
future.

The storm, he said, took what was for many a rather abstract and distant idea
of global warming and turned it into something that was "tangible and con-
crete and scary. Because we know that we should expect more events like Sandy
in a world where there are hotter temperatures, warmer oceans, and thermal
expansion."

After Sandy, Klinenberg began working to advance collaborative research and
design that could make cities and the built environment more resilient against
climate change. He became research director for a new federal project called
Rebuild by Design (*www.rebuildbydesign.org*), a design competition launched

---

Box 12.1

One such initiative is the Hunts Point Lifelines Project in the South
Bronx in New York City. Located on a square-mile peninsula surrounded
by water, Hunts Point serves as the hub of the food supply for 25 million
people in the northeast section of the country, housing produce, fish, and
meat markets while providing over 10,000 jobs to the region. Ironically,
Klinenberg describes the surrounding neighborhood as a true example of
health disparities: residents of Hunts Point are located in one of the poorest
congressional districts in the United States, with some of the highest rates
of asthma and diabetes in New York and with little access to fresh food from
the wholesale markets.

Although Hurricane Sandy spared much of Hunts Point from water
damage, the area is extremely vulnerable to flooding and "has been threatened by climate change in all kinds of really difficult ways." According to
Klinenberg, the Hunts Point facilities are old and its antiquated power grid
and refrigeration systems are fragile. With $20 million in funding from the
federal government, the Hunts Point Lifelines Project coordinated through
Rebuild by Design proposed four "lifelines" to help address these issues,
with ideas that ranged from flood protection and job creation to maritime
emergency supply lines to low-cost, low-carbon cooling plants. After a
year-long community engagement project, and an additional $25 million
in funding from the city, the project has identified two areas for feasibility
studies: flood risk reduction and resilient energy systems.

by the U.S. Department of Housing and Urban Development in partnership with nonprofits and the philanthropic sector in response to Hurricane Sandy. The overarching goal of the project was to help communities respond, prepare, and be resilient when confronted with natural challenges. Rebuild by Design's Hurricane Sandy Design Competition changed the way the federal government responded to disaster, and became the model now used in other regions to prepare communities for future uncertainties and help them coordinate resilience strategies.

Through Rebuild by Design, Klinenberg didn't attempt to rebuild New York City or parts of New Jersey damaged by the storm. Rather, he said, Rebuild by Design helped communities and neighborhoods embrace resilience-building projects "in anticipation of the kind of weather that is coming, and the kind of threats that are coming" (Box 12.1).

Klinenberg concludes, "We are being forced to reckon with what it's like to live in these new conditions. We're effectively living in a new ecology now. The planet works differently than it used to."

The Health System Infrastructure: Vulnerable

Klinenberg challenged everyone to think about the significance of health system infrastructures and how vulnerable the delivery of health care can be when a crisis hits. He pointed out that during Hurricane Sandy, hospitals throughout New York City and the region lost power and many didn't have adequate backup systems. He advocates a long-term study of the health impacts of the storm and the people most affected by interruption of care. "We are entering into a world where we're going to be dealing with those situations more often."

Klinenberg recently edited a collection of essays about how cities and nations are trying to adapt to emerging climate change problems. In Buenos Aires, for example, rapid urban development and rising energy consumption have taxed the local power grid beyond capacity; the Argentinean capital is working to prevent blackouts during summer heatwaves through initiatives that curb electricity consumption and incentivize local companies to improve energy efficiency.[4]

Though he pointed out that the United States is "extraordinarily advantaged" when it comes to having resources to deal with threats of climate change, Klinenberg argued that this does not mean these systems are always protected. "We are vulnerable in so many ways," he said. "It's extraordinary to think about the disruption of health care from extreme weather events. It's time for people

[4] For more information, see "The Impact of Climate Change on Health and Equity," *www.rwjf.org/en/culture-of-health/2016/06/what_does_climatech.html*.

who are working on health all the time, and investing in better health systems, to take this issue seriously. It cannot be avoided."

Reflections on Research

Within its Culture of Health framework, RWJF not only recognizes the serious health consequences of climate change but also highlights the need for community resilience, preparedness, and stewardship. Toward this goal, RWJF supports related research and policy initiatives in four key areas:[5]

- **Strengthening community resilience.** The Foundation joined with The Gulf Research program of the National Academies of Sciences, Engineering, and Medicine to establish a $10 million grants initiative to fund projects that enhance the science and practice of coastal community resilience in the Gulf of Mexico region.

  The research projects will: highlight connections between community resilience and health; explore health, social, environmental, and economic impacts of disasters and other environmental stressors; and inform strategies to address these challenges in Gulf communities. The projects will not focus on infrastructure needs or the built environments, which are being targeted by many resilience-focused programs; rather, this program supports the study of the human dynamics (physical and mental health, social cohesiveness, and social and economic well-being) that influence a community's ability to respond to adverse events.
- **Designing healthy communities.** With support from RWJF and the Pew Charitable Trusts, the Minnesota Department of Health is creating a toolkit to help public health departments, city planners, and others conduct health impact assessments on proposed climate change projects and policies.[6]
- **Ensuring emergency preparedness and response.** In the aftermath of Hurricane Sandy, RWJF supported a nonprofit organization called Sustainable Jersey (*www.sustainablejersey.com*) that developed action plans for local municipalities to help them confront climate change impacts. With these plans in place, local communities are better prepared to respond to short-term emergencies caused by extreme heat, drought, and flooding and to improve their community's overall resiliency.

---

[5] For more information, see "The Impact of Climate Change on Health and Equity," *www.rwjf. org/en/culture-of-health/2016/06/what_does_climatech.html*.

[6] Minnesota Department of Health, Health Impact Assessment Reports, *www.health.state.mn.us/ divs/hia/reports.html*.

- **Encouraging environmental stewardship.** With a grant from RWJF, an international organization called Health Care Without Harm (*www.noharm-uscanada.org*) has identified a series of environmentally sound practices and policies that can help hospitals and doctors' offices reduce their environmental footprint and protect the health and safety of patients and health care workers. Key practices, for instance, include removing harmful toxins and reducing waste.

According to Plough's hopeful assessment, "tackling the effects of climate change requires that leaders from all sectors of a community work together, which can lead to better health, stronger communities, and greater equity in health and well-being. That's a triple win."

Reflections on Policy and Practice

Despite the well-documented impacts of climate change around the globe, there is not yet a shared value around this issue, which clearly baffled the experts and members of the audience. As Klinenberg asked: "How do you persuade people who don't believe in science to believe in science?"

McCormick and Rudolph both noted that while climate change is a clear threat to health, action that reverses or lessens damaging environmental practices presents real health opportunities. Consider climate change transformations to energy, agriculture, and transportation industries:

- Moving to clean, renewable energy would reduce greenhouse gas emissions and air pollution that cause asthma and heart disease.
- In agriculture, reducing meat consumption and improving access to local, sustainably produced fruits and vegetables would reduce many chronic diseases, increase food security, and reduce methane emissions and carbon pollution.
- Within the transportation industry, improving public transit and biking and walking infrastructures would increase physical activity, help decrease many diseases associated with sedentary lifestyles, and reduce greenhouse gas emissions.

Reflecting on this climate change health paradox, Rudolph said, "Climate action presents remarkable health opportunities, too."

But McCormick and Rudolph also described a systematic and well-funded effort to sow doubt about climate change in the minds of the public, efforts that work against the opportunities for the health benefits they envision. They said powerful institutions were using their influence to maintain the country's addiction to fossil fuel and presenting experts who questioned whether there are enough data to substantiate the dangers. Rudolph reminded the audience that this paralleled what happened with tobacco, when the tobacco industry tried to deny that smoking caused diseases before public health, scientific evidence, and organizations like RWJF successfully intervened and the public began to respond.[7] History appears to be repeating itself, they said.

Klinenberg saw an even bigger challenge: How do you make climate change real and urgent? Ticking off a lineup of health and environment issues that he said are always given priority over climate change—universal access to health care, obesity, lead in the water, unemployment—Klinenberg issued a dire warning: "The paradox is, if we wait until climate change is the most important thing, it's too late."

From Urgency to Equity: The World in Relationship to Others

As people who care about health, we have to make sure that the solutions we choose for climate change are implemented with a health and equity lens.
—Linda Rudolph

Rudolph agreed that it is important to convince people around the world that climate change is an urgent matter. But, she pointed out, a paradox of climate change is that it can seem overwhelming to fully consider its potentially catastrophic consequences. One of the challenges, she said, is to help policymakers understand and tackle climate change in manageable steps, to recognize that "there is a lot that we can do at every level of government and in our own communities to address this."

During a spirited question-and-answer session, audience members pondered the meaning of equity in relation to climate change and the Culture of Health. Several called for a fundamental shift in how we view the world and our relationship to one another and to our natural resources. Rudolph, for one, believes strongly in the "aspect of intergenerational equity" embedded in climate change discussions. She argued: "We're essentially mortgaging the future of our children in terms of the future impacts of climate change with what kinds of choices we're making now, or not making, as the case may be. We are risking a discontinuity in human survival because of the extent to which we are putting our ecosystems at risk."

---

[7] For more than 25 years, RWJF has been on the front lines of the battle against the harm caused by tobacco products, the largest cause of preventable death in the nation. For more information, see *www.rwjf.org/en/library/articles-and-news/2016/05/robert-wood-johnson-foundation-statement-on-fda-rule-to-further.html*.

Discussions also focused on the value of building and developing communities in ways that are sustainable and resilient and help improve health and well-being. Initiatives that have co-benefits for health and the environment should be more widely promoted, Klinenberg said, such as the design of neighborhoods with more green spaces and parks to promote physical activity (issues discussed more fully in Chapter 10, *Building Healthy Cities*). A core principle of Rebuild by Design, he said, is that "we should always look for projects that will not just protect us from an acute event, but will also improve the health and well-being of communities every day. You should get multiple benefits out of every design."

Rudolph reviewed California's efforts to be a leader in creating climate change policies that not only set the tone for the rest of the nation but work to integrate public health, equity, and health in all policy frameworks; the state's transportation agency, for instance, now has health in its mission statement.

How to Frame the Story of Climate Change

Integrating climate change and health may be very effective in the long run, most seemed to agree, because health is a more prominent social issue and resonates with people on a personal level. But when it comes to issues of sustainability and resilience, some questioned how to even begin the conversation and integration process.

Take climate change and emergency preparedness, particularly in rural areas. "What words do you use?" said Dennis Andrulis, PhD, associate professor at the University of Texas School of Public Health, who has over 30 years of experience in health care research and policy focused on vulnerable populations, their providers, and their communities. "If you use 'climate change' or 'emergency preparedness' in most quarters, the terms are not tailored to the circumstances, nor is the language familiar to them."

Andrulis said he relies on data to help raise involvement, awareness, and the "likelihood of people buying in." For instance, he draws from several data sources to document climate-related events like fire, hurricanes, and floods, and then integrates data with leading social determinants and health measures such as self-reported health, obesity, poverty, diversity and access to health care. "When you mapped these determinants with the events, you could actually identify specific areas that are hit with what we call 'perfect storms.'"

Using data and mapping can also make people more aware of how climate change impacts everyone around them—even if they had not previously made the connection with local businesses, employment opportunities, and the economic health of the area. When it's clear that climate change impacts the way people make their living and earn money, "that is when they may perk up their ears," Andrulis said.

The process is daunting, McCormick agreed. "Your comments very much remind me of a phrase that's something like, 'Climate change is generated globally but experienced locally.'" And then McCormick drew from her documentary filmmaking expertise to implore people to talk about climate change by simply telling stories. Tell stories and frame stories, she said, in ways that encourage people to pay attention, to have characters that communities care about. In crafting this increasingly important story, she argued that drawing on health consequences is not only an accurate storytelling framework but an excellent way to create a sense of multigenerational urgency around climate change. Ultimately, "when you use the health implications of climate change to help frame it, it's no longer this 'thing' that affects somebody else at some other time in some other place. It's something that affects me, or my grandmother, or my child."

In closing, Rudolph provided a revised vision for the Culture of Health, where planetary health and climate change encircle its Action Framework. Why? Because civilization cannot exist without the ability to drink clean water, breathe clean air, grow sufficient amounts of nutritious food, and live in safe housing that isn't destroyed by wind and water. And because, all three experts agreed, we simply can't have an equitable Culture of Health without acknowledging that we live on a planet that must sustain us. It is, they agreed, the most profound challenge humanity has ever faced.

PART FIVE

INNOVATING TO BUILD
A CULTURE OF HEALTH

Though the scope of work described in the previous section is broad and deep, creative cross-disciplinary thinkers are not stopping there. Across the country, they are testing novel solutions and implementing innovations that represent intriguing approaches to doing business, and just may help build better health for all. *Innovating to Build a Culture of Health* looks at a few of those approaches, which collectively are broadening our thinking and allowing us to push forward, inspired by a deepening belief that progress is possible. All are young attempts to realize long-term change.

We present them not as strategies we endorse, because they are mostly too new for that, or to encourage other jurisdictions to implement them. Rather, the intent is to demonstrate that a Culture of Health is a "big tent" that welcomes many ideas from many sectors—the initiatives featured here involve two private investment firms, an umbrella community organization, classroom teachers, a city health department, a policy organization, and a philanthropic organization. Their activities are not connected to one another, but their convergence at this moment in time perhaps reflects a growing consensus that creating a Culture of Health is this country's best, or perhaps only, shot at achieving well-being or even surviving as a civil society. They bring to life some key elements of that effort: collaboration, application of knowledge to action, and engagement of people on the front line.

Public, Private, Nonprofit Partnership: A Case Study of Social Impact Bonds looks at a financing model designed to attract private investors into human capital and social service programs. *Forward in Baltimore: Illuminating the Possible, Achieving the Potential* takes a closer look at efforts to change a city that face great challenges, but has tremendous potential, as well as the use of the Genuine Progress Indicator, adopted in Maryland in 2010. Finally, *A Look Inside the Robert Wood Johnson Foundation* offers thoughtful reflections from RWJF staff on how the Foundation itself has changed through its journey into a Culture of Health. While acknowledging how inequities continue to damage well-being, the concluding chapter offers an appreciation of the work that is underway and sounds a call to action for all that remains to be done.

Public, Private, Nonprofit Partnership

A Case Study of Social Impact Bonds

CHRIS ELLIS, SOCIAL INNOVATION STRATEGIST, FOURTH ECONOMY
CONSULTING, AND FORMER PARTNERSHIP DIRECTOR FOR EARLY
LEARNING OUTCOMES, UNITED WAY OF SALT LAKE

ANDREA PHILLIPS, MPP, FOUNDER AND MANAGING PARTNER, MAYCOMB
CAPITAL, AND FORMER VICE PRESIDENT, URBAN INVESTMENT GROUP
OF GOLDMAN SACHS

JOHN ROMAN, PHD, SENIOR FELLOW, NORC AT THE UNIVERSITY
OF CHICAGO, AND FORMER SENIOR FELLOW, URBAN INSTITUTE

Can the delivery of quality social services create returns for private investors? Social impact bonds are trying to answer that question. Incubated in the United Kingdom in 2010 as a way of financing programs to reduce recidivism among offenders, social impact bonds have been scaled to 15 countries, across 60 projects by June 2016. The first social impact bond in the United States was executed in August 2012.

Social impact bonds—a financial tool in which private investment dollars lend capital to finance the expansion of human, health, and social service programs that work—tap into core aspects of building a Culture of Health for all Americans. They require a new type of relationships among private investors, government agencies, social service providers, and evaluators. They rest on the provision of high-quality social programs delivered at enough scale to make a broad impact. They are not quick fixes; they rely instead on solid commitment of multiple actors over time.

Three panelists representing an investment firm, an umbrella social services agency, and an evaluation organization explored how Salt Lake City used a social impact bond to expand access to high-quality early childhood education.

Social Impact Bonds: What They Are and How They Work

A social impact bond is not a bond. It is a working capital loan against the proceeds of a pay-for-success contract."—Andrea Phillips

Social impact bonds—also known as pay-for-success financings or outcomes-based financings—have emerged as a tool for government to fund what works and improve outcomes for disadvantaged communities. In a social impact bond, private investment firms provide upfront working capital to help finance the expansion of a social service to a community. Investors are repaid only if the program achieves outcomes specified in the contract. Social impact bonds rest on the belief that prevention and early intervention programs yield both human and financial benefits—they are a triple-win for governments, service providers, and communities.

Investors provide the necessary working capital to bridge the gap between the time when services are provided and the time when the savings that generate repayment are realized. They also take on the risk of impact (i.e., the chance that the social intervention may not produce results in the community).

"Impact investments aim to generate financial returns while simultaneously driving towards a very intentional social impact," says Andrea Phillips. "These social impact bond opportunities are underwritten as any other loan would be, with additional attention paid to social impact."

Essential actors in a social impact bond relationship are:

- A government agency wanting to address a significant social issue such as homelessness, recidivism, or early childhood development
- A private investor willing to front funds for an intervention to address the issue
- An intermediary organization able to sign the loan agreement, contract with service providers, oversee the initiative, and repay the investor
- One or more community-based organizations with proven interventions and the capacity to deliver the services
- An evaluator prepared to conduct a rigorous study of service outcomes and impacts.

This arrangement among multiple stakeholders aligns incentives and holds everyone accountable for results. Government agencies, service providers, and evaluators come together, with the shared goal of achieving broader impact than each could achieve on its own. Impact investments like these have more typically been utilized to finance brick-and-mortar projects that revitalize communities such as local health centers and mixed-income housing. For example, Goldman Sachs has committed more than $5 billion in impact investments such as these since 2001.

Sharing Risk

A core feature of social impact bonds is shared risk, or "pay for success." This notion of risk is new and at times unusual for social service and government agencies whose historical contractual relationships have been and are still generally based on reimbursement for services rendered.

Standard fee-for-service contracts may reduce risk, but they have limitations. They usually pay based on activity measures such as number of people served and types of services provided. While these measures are essential for active program management, they provide little information about whether the ultimate outcomes are achieved and do not directly address the quality of the services delivered.

When there is a large gap between the time during which a service is delivered and the time when government savings or future benefits are accrued from the provision of effective services, an outcomes-based contract may be helpful. For instance, savings and/or future benefits from improved preventive health care, stable housing, or reduced recidivism are usually not available until long after the costs of delivering these services have been incurred.

"Most service providers don't have the financial wherewithal to take on all the risk of these pay-for-success contracts," says Phillips. "That's what the financial markets do all the time."

Paying for Outcomes and Impacts

When payment is contingent on performance, all stakeholders develop a laser-like focus on the outcomes and impacts. Defining expected targeted outcomes—performance metrics to be attained—and anticipated impacts—changes in behaviors or circumstances to be realized—entails both cooperation and innovation among government, private investors, intermediary agencies, and evaluators.

Considerations include: How long should investors wait for outcomes and impacts? What is a fair interest rate? What are reasonable outcomes and impacts to expect from service providers? How will we know if those have been achieved?

"There is room for negotiation in there," says Phillips. "The expected returns on these deals for the senior investor have been mid-to-high single digits. The terms of these deals and the appetite for typical investors is probably five to eight years."

To offset the full burden of risk, many impact investors seek a level of "de-risking" or credit enhancement in each investment. Typical of other investments, these credit enhancements may include a partial principal guarantee from a phil-anthropic organization or a secondary investor with more risk appetite.

Theory Meets Practice: Social Impact Bonds in Salt Lake City

Studies and experience have shown that high-quality early childhood educa-tion programs lead to improved academic and emotional development, and that these benefits last. Giving a child a solid foundation early in life also saves money in later remedial, special education, and other costs.

Context: A Preschool Program in the Right Place at the Right Time

In the early 2000s, the Granite School District in Salt Lake City sought to ex-pand its Utah High Quality Preschool Program. A request for federal funds for this purpose was approved and the ensuing program enhancements resulted in strong outcomes for all children, but especially for the low-income children who attended the program.

"We followed those kids when they were in third and fourth grade, and found that the achievement gap between these low-income kids and their more afflu-ent peers was effectively closed," says Chris Ellis.

The school district brought to the partnership table, therefore, a program with a solid track record of documented success over a period of years and a desire to expand its reach by recruiting more children. The United Way brought a con-sortium of business, government, evaluation, and nonprofit leaders with a his-tory of working together for the Salt Lake community. Goldman Sachs and J. B. Pritzker brought money and a willingness to risk it on investments in children.

Enter Social Impact Bonds

Discussions with Goldman Sachs began in 2010, which is the first year social impact bonds appeared on the policy and financing horizon in the United States. According to Phillips, "The first thing we asked was 'How do we know that you are going to achieve the impacts you need to achieve that will allow the contract to repay us?' Achieving these goals drives both the social impact and repayment of the loan."

The team on the ground in Salt Lake City had answers. They were able to produce several years of outcome data from evaluations of the preschool program, describe and share its curriculum, and offer detailed projections about expansion plans. Importantly, the team also demonstrated a shared vision and cohesive management and leadership capacity.

By June 2013, officials at United Way of Salt Lake had negotiated $7 million in private-sector loans, to be repaid with interest from savings realized by reduced costs of special education services attributed to the Utah High Quality Preschool Program.

With the start of the 2013-14 school year, Utah's "Pay-for-Success" program became the country's first social impact bond for early childhood services. It financed an expansion of the Utah High Quality Preschool Program to serve 3,500 new children recruited in five cohorts. There were no upfront costs to taxpayers.

Key actors at the outset of Pay-for-Success were:

- Government: State and county officials
- Investors: Goldman Sachs (the primary investor, $4.6 million loan); J. B. Pritzker (secondary investor, $2.4 million loan)
- Intermediary: United Way of Salt Lake
- Service provider: Granite School District
- Evaluator: Utah State University

Chris Ellis recalls, "We saw this as an opportunity to further our collective impact work. We played the backbone role, helping facilitate and align partnerships at schools, at system levels and with other preschool providers."

In the 2013–14 school year, 595 low-income children entered the preschool program. All 595 children were screened using the Peabody Picture Vocabulary Test. Some 110 were identified through screening as likely to require special education services while in grade school.

Evaluators from Utah State University are tracking these 110 children through sixth grade to determine whether they utilize special education services, and for how long. No one from the preschool program, the United Way, or Goldman Sachs knows which children are being tracked.

Following the Money

By 2015, early findings from the evaluator suggested that the preschool program and the Pay-for-Success financing strategy were working. Of the 110 children identified as likely to need special education in grade school, only one went on to use those services in kindergarten.

With that milestone, investors were due their first repayment, the first such payment for a social impact bond in the United States. Through formulas used to determine the cost of special education services avoided, savings were determined to be $281,550 in the first year, or $2,607 per child[1] for children served by the program during its first year. These savings generated a payment to investors of about $267,000.[2] If performance continues as expected, estimated savings to the State of Utah for the first cohort of children would exceed $1 million through 12th grade.[3]

Under the Pay-for-Success contract with the State of Utah, investors receive 95 percent of state savings in special education costs until the investments are repaid with interest.[4] The base interest rate on the loan is 5 percent.[5] Thereafter, Goldman Sachs and Pritzker will receive "success fees" until the children complete sixth grade or until the return is 7.25 percent. Savings after that time will accrue to the state and school districts.[6] Chris Ellis recalled, "Once the rest of the partnerships were established, all we needed was an agency to repay the loan investment based on the success of the program for cohorts 2–5. We figured that the government made the most sense and securing their participation would be fairly straightforward. This, however, proved to be a complex process."

Initial efforts to pass state legislation to repay investors did not succeed. To keep Pay-for-Success on track, therefore, the board of directors of the United Way of Salt Lake set aside $1 million and Salt Lake County set aside $350,000 to repay investors for the first cohort of children.

In the next year, with passage of HB96: the Utah School Readiness Initiative in March 2014, the Utah State Legislature allocated funds for repayment of investor loans for the remaining four cohorts of children. The Act also allows a newly established School Readiness Board to enter into Pay-for-Success contracts with private investors on behalf of the state, and authorizes other expansions of early childhood education throughout the state. "We were expanding access to proven quality programs and through the legislation were able to change the conversation in Utah around early childhood education," said Ellis.

---

[1] www.ssir.org/articles/entry/pay_for_success_is_working_in_utah

[2] www.sltrib.com/home/3032598-155/preschool-paying-off-for-goldman-sachs

[3] www.goldmansachs.com/what-we-do/investing-and-lending/impact-investing/case-studies/sib-slc-fact-sheet.pdf

[4] www.sltrib.com/home/3032598-155/preschool-paying-off-for-goldman-sachs

[5] www.hceconomics.uchicago.edu/sites/default/files/file_uploads/SIB-RBFFact_SheetUtahVersion.pdf

[6] www.hceconomics.uchicago.edu/sites/default/files/file_uploads/SIB-RBFFact_SheetUtahVersion.pdf

Reflections

I think there is a little myopia about raising private capital to help govern-
ment do the things it doesn't do, and one of the things I get asked is, "Why
doesn't government just do these things?"—John Roman

The experience in Utah is encouraging, but social impact bonds are new and
many questions remain unresolved.[7] Utah's experience illuminates these questions and raises other issues that warrant further exploration.

Why Has Uptake Been Slow?

As of March 2016, Goldman Sachs had executed four social impact bond investments. Executing the contract in Utah, which was especially well positioned to
use this approach, took three years.

What is a reasonable time line for developing a social impact bond or
outcomes-based financing? Will experience lead to shorter time lines? What
accounts for a slow uptake in interest?

Government agencies and investment firms are cautious about doing business in such a fundamentally different way. Some point to government as a major
source of bottleneck and others point to the investment firms.

John Roman holds that there are high-net-worth individuals, venture capi-
talists, and private investment firms "who are looking for investments like this
and want to invest in good works." He asks why government agencies in particular seem reticent to get involved in these transactions. "We are talking about
100 percent reduction in their risk, and the government says 'No, thank you.'"

There are reasons for government hesitancy. City and county officials, those
most likely to pursue social impact bonds, are not necessarily familiar with
the language and intricacies of private investment. In addition, public entities
responsible for repaying the loans must feel confident that the programs they
propose are well developed and are backed by enough of the "right kind" of
evidence.

Higher levels of government impose multiple regulatory and reporting
requirements on city and county government agencies, and those requirements have to be considered. "The good news is there is a lot of work going on

---

[7] For example, some have challenged use of the Peabody Picture Vocabulary test as an appropriate method of screening children for special education needs. See *www.nytimes.com/2015/11/04/
business/dealbook/did-goldman-make-the-grade.html?_r=0* for this discussion and *www.nytimes.com/
2015/11/14/business/dealbook/why-social-impact-bonds-still-have-promise.html*.

in Washington to get the federal government to okay these types of structures," says Phillips.

Louise Cohen, MPH, CEO of the Primary Care Development Corporation and moderator of the panel, asked why investors weren't flocking to opportunities that purport to offer "high-digit" return on investments in proven social programs. In response, Andrea Phillips explained that "the deals are hard to do because they ask government and other stakeholders to do business in a new way. But with 60 deals done globally, we believe we are on the cusp of seeing more standardization and simplification. I'm cautiously optimistic that these efficiencies will lead to real growth of this nascent market."

How Much Evidence Is Enough Evidence?

Investors seeking reassurance that they will be repaid understandably favor programs with long track records of outcomes and impacts. But how much evidence is enough? How often do proven programs have to re-prove their effectiveness? Are investors open to financing less mature programs that show promise? Those questions have not been answered.

Cohen argues that government agencies use evidence-based interventions that yield strong outcomes "all the time." The bigger challenge, she maintains, is scaling an innovative approach that evidence has shown to work in a "boutique" setting. How seriously would private investors consider investing in one of these programs without needing a new randomized controlled trial?

Phillips suggests an alternative to asking investors to support these younger but promising interventions. "I do think that is a great role for philanthropy, as an angel investor in the early stages of innovation."

At the other end of the evidence spectrum, some programs—Nurse-Family Partnership for one—have decades of solid evidence behind them demonstrating their long-term impacts and cost savings. Do they need yet more evidence to establish their value? Perhaps the evaluation should examine the financing mechanism rather than the intervention.

"From where we sit as investors, we are looking for a contract that clearly defines the outcomes we expect and how we will know if we got there," says Phillips. "Investors will look at prior evaluations and historical data to assess the likelihood of achieving the agreed-upon outcomes."

There is not a simple or single way to address these challenges. Decisions about whether to propose or finance a program for a social impact bond require shared confidence that at some future date there will be consensus about whether the intervention unfolded as it was supposed to and whether it achieved the intended outcomes.

Arriving at that shared confidence may entail negotiating an acceptable middle ground. The city of Chicago, for example, aimed to use its social impact bond to increase high school graduation rates, but investors wanted a more immediate repayment trigger. The city, the school district, and the investors ultimately agreed on three benchmarks—kindergarten readiness, third-grade reading, and decreased rates of special education usage—which, taken together, would be strong enough indicators of future high school graduation.

In the case of Utah's preschool program, it was not hard for all partners to agree on the big goal—keeping young children in Utah on track at school. The question then became how to measure progress to reach consensus on whether that happened.

How Big Is Big Enough? What Is Adequate Scale?

What does it mean to go to scale? Salt Lake City's Pay-for-Success, for example, increased participation in quality preschool programs, eliminated the 400-child waiting list for early childhood services in Salt Lake, and allowed new children to be recruited. It also expanded from the Granite School District to one additional district, two private providers, a charter school, and one nonprofit organization. Is that a reasonable expectation for one social impact bond? Does this expansion "count" as scale?

Roman believes that, with good data, there are ways to answer those questions. He characterizes social impact bonds as "forcing mechanisms" that promote both scaling and quality improvement. Within evaluations of stable programs trying to expand their reach, "there also tends to be a component that examines, 'Are we implementing with fidelity?' and 'Are there subgroups for whom this works better?'"

Ellis took a broad perspective. He noted that the social impact bond had prompted the first expansion of early education services, which in turn prompted state legislation in Utah that added yet more capacity and provided a stable source of funding over time. Importantly, this experience also engendered significant changes in how stakeholders talk about early childhood education.

"We have seen that new grants are improving quality around the state. I don't know if social impact bonds alone are going to be the strategy that allows us to meet the commitment we have to all children, but the bonds have been able to catalyze more conversations about early childhood education," he said. "The providers are not talking only about programmatic-level outcomes. They are also talking about how what they are doing aligns with the broader atmosphere around early childhood education."

Can the System Be Gamed?

Is there potential for manipulating an intervention to skew results? Are there protections against paying or otherwise coercing people to engage in a desired behavior, thereby falsely suggesting that the social intervention reached its intended outcomes?

Roman notes that, while "there is a lot of pressure for me to put my finger on the dial toward a particular outcome," the partnership structure of social impact bonds reduces the likelihood that will happen. The participation of multiple partners in intensive contract negotiations surfaces and clarifies the incentives that drive each partner to participate. This means the intervention takes on a collective nature. As Roman puts it, "This is the only place in governance where there is a collective understanding of other people's incentives, and if we want to scale the use of evidence, having that collective among all the partners is absolutely critical."

What Attributes of a Community Suggest Success?

Phillips noted several characteristics investors value in deciding whether to invest in community financing: a group of people capable of implementing the project, a system with capacity to scale, a management team with depth, and sound systems of performance management and professional development. "This is similar to what we consider with any type of investment. We are not trying to micromanage what is happening on the ground. We ask the service providers to explain to us what the core principles of the program are and how they have delivered the outcomes in the past. Then, they can have nimbleness around that."

Investors also look for reassurance as to the creditworthiness of the proposed contract. Two, three, or even five years down the road, will the government in fact repay the loan? The issue of future appropriation is not unique to social impact bonds but is a challenge faced in many government contracts. Particularly in this nascent phase of the social impact bond market, this is a risk that investors acknowledge and for which they have developed strategies such as legislative action, contractual language, and more.

Social impact bonds in the United States are little more than four years old. Only a handful of contracts have been executed, and, although it is too early to be certain whether this approach to growing and improving social services will endure, early results show strong signs of success. Within the context of building a Culture of Health, a strategy in which public, nonprofit, and private-sector partners collaborate and put their financial and programmatic assets on the table deserves a full and fair test.

Forward in Baltimore

Illuminating the Possible, Achieving the Potential

LEW DALY, DIRECTOR OF POLICY AND RESEARCH, DEMOS

LEANA S. WEN, MD, MSC, COMMISSIONER OF HEALTH, BALTIMORE CITY

With a population of 623,000, Baltimore is a city of neighborhoods and history. It is home to Johns Hopkins University, the Baltimore Orioles, the Baltimore Symphony, the Inner Harbor, and the National Aquarium. Edgar Allan Poe, Frederick Douglass, Babe Ruth, and Billie Holiday resided in the city at one time or another, and Francis Scott Key wrote *The Star Spangled Banner* there. Downtown Baltimore is experiencing an influx of young professionals drawn by an increasingly vibrant restaurant and nightlife scene and housing that is inexpensive in comparison with many large cities.

At the same time, Baltimore crime rates are higher than the national average and 2015 saw 344 homicides—a record-setting rate of 55 per 100,000 residents. That year, of course, included the April 19 death of Freddie Gray while in police custody and the unrest that followed. Afterwards, killings climbed steeply. There had been a total of 58 homicides from January through mid-April, but May brought 42 more—the worst month in decades—topped by 45 in July, with a monthly average of 31 for the rest of the year. Blacks, who make up 63 percent of the population, accounted for 93 percent of homicide victims.[1] Years of complaints by black residents about targeted police abuse were corroborated by a U.S. Justice Department report on the Baltimore Police Department released in August 2016.

Like many cities Baltimore has great strengths, great challenges, and great potential. As such it can be viewed as something of a microcosm of American

---

[1] Crime statistics reported by the *New York Times* on January 15, 2016, in "The Numbers Behind Baltimore's Record Year in Homicides," *www.nytimes.com/interactive/2016/01/14/us/Baltimore-homicides-record.html*.

urban life and the difficulties inherent in weaving a Culture of Health into the thick fabric of a struggling but optimistic city. As we examine problem-solving innovations around the country in this section, Baltimore certainly warrants a closer look.

In contrast to the often negative picture of Baltimore evident in news reports, the contributors to this chapter offered a sense of hope that one city, in one state, can make a difference in the health of its people through the efforts of researchers, public officials, practitioners, and, most importantly, its own people working day to day to address inequity and—wittingly or not—build a Culture of Health for all its residents.

Pushing Back: The Role of Public Health in a City in Flux

We strongly believe it's the role of public health to push back ... In public health we are delivering the services to level the playing field of inequality.—Leana Wen

Formed in 1793, the Baltimore City Health Department is the country's oldest continuously operating health department. In January 2015, Mayor Stephanie Rawlings-Blake appointed Dr. Leana S. Wen, an emergency physician and patient and community advocate, as Baltimore City Health Commissioner.

After Freddie Gray's death, images of the city's burned and looted pharmacies splashed across the Internet, TV screens, and newspapers. In her job as commissioner, Wen immediately grasped the public health need resulting from the 13 ruined pharmacies: hundreds of seniors—many in wheelchairs, oxygen-dependent, unable to access another store outside their neighborhood—were now without vital medications. Frantic calls came in to the health department: a woman who was going to stop eating until she could get her insulin; people so short of breath as a result of running out of their inhalers that the department called ambulances to take them to a hospital.

This situation illustrates the interweaving of health and health care in the fabric of city life. "You can't just look at the violence that occurred and talk about it being a criminal justice problem without also thinking about the individuals who this has most affected," said Wen. The rioting and looting youth cannot be seen only as perpetrators of violence without acknowledging that they themselves are victims of violence, crime, intergenerational poverty, and the "deep disparities" that result. Wen noted that, as a child, Freddie Gray was lead-poisoned and, thus, vulnerable to lifelong effects on learning ability and physical, mental, social, and emotional health.

But not all of the stories out of Baltimore are so distressing and Wen believes it is time to hear "some good stories" about what is happening in public health in the city. Wen shared three examples of public health pushing back and helping to level the field in Baltimore by providing the supports needed to further the health of its residents:

- In 2009, Baltimore had one of the highest rates of infant mortality in the country, on par with Syria, according to Wen. The Baltimore Health Department and the Family League of Baltimore, more than 150 donors, public agencies, health providers, home visiting programs, and community, academic, and national partners launched B'more for Healthy Babies (*www.healthybabiesbaltimore.com*) that year. A full complement of programs (addressing safe sleep, baby basics, teen pregnancy prevention, smoking, prenatal care, substance-exposed pregnancies, and other key issues) is offered to fulfill the vision that "all of Baltimore's babies are born at a healthy weight, full term, and ready to thrive in healthy families."

  Now, seven years since B'more's launch, reported Wen, sleep-related infant deaths are down by half. The overall infant mortality rate decreased by 38 percent between 2009 and 2015, with the rate for black infants declining by almost 50 percent.[2] In addition, said Wen, though not an initial focus of the program, teen birth rates have fallen by 36 percent.

  Not only does this affect the baby whose life is saved, said Wen, "which is already incredible," but it improves educational outcomes, which later will reduce family violence, and ultimately "cut off that cycle of intergenerational poverty and violence and trauma that otherwise plagues us . . . When we look to see what it is that public health can do, that is what an upstream approach can do to save lives."

- Safe Streets (*www.health.baltimorecity.gov/safestreets*), a violence-prevention program operated by the Baltimore City Health Department, hires individuals known in their community—many who are former gang members or drug dealers, or have recently been released from incarceration—to walk the streets and interrupt conflict and violence where they see it. In 2014 Safe Streets violence interrupters intervened in 880 conflicts, of which 80 percent were considered to be likely or very likely to result in gun violence.

---

[2] Figures from B'more for Healthy Babies website at *www.healthybabiesbaltimore.com/news-and-events/news/2016/10/05/infant-mortality-in-baltimore-city-down-to-a-record-low*

A great deal of public money is spent on police work, the criminal justice system, and incarceration, Wen pointed out, yet little is spent on prevention. "The face of prevention is always hard to describe because you can't see it. You can see the person shot, you can see the person who died from a heart attack. You can't see the person in whom we prevented injury and disease. That is the job that we have in public health."

Telling the stories of efforts that work, like Safe Streets, helps both to change the conversation, and to make resources available to hire the very people who can actually do the needed work, stressed Wen: "We don't see our citizens as problems. We see them as solutions to every problem. They are partners to everything that we do."

- The Baltimore City Health Department has launched "one of the most aggressive overdose prevention and treatment programs[3] in the country[4]," said Wen. More people die of overdoses than from homicide in Baltimore.[5]

Wen issued a blanket prescription for naloxone, the antidote medication for opioid overdose, for all Baltimore residents so that everyone can have the drug available to save a life. As of September 2016, the Health Department had trained nearly 15,000 people in its use, including police officers. In the first month carrying naloxone, officers used it to save the lives of four people. Citizens and other laypeople have used naloxone to save over 500 lives in Baltimore.

The opioid addiction crisis requires a host of solutions—medication, psychosocial support, long-term recovery programs, and so on[6]—but the widespread availability of naloxone is a start. Building on that start means implementing a broader view of public health like the view articulated by Wen: "This is what we do in public health. We look at the problem, find innovative solutions, and call the problem as we see it. We cannot be afraid to say that mass incarceration is a public health issue, that racism is a public health issue; that it's our policies of longtime discrimination and structural racism that have led us to the disparities in Baltimore and elsewhere."

---

[3] www.health.baltimorecity.gov/opioid-overdose/baltimore-city-overdose-prevention-and-response-information

[4] www.usatoday.com/story/news/health/2016/03/04/doctor-wants-overdose-antidote-every-medicine-cabinet/81291850/

[5] www.npr.org/sections/health-shots/2015/04/10/396884295/a-life-saving-medication-that-my-patient-didn-t-get

[6] www.washingtonpost.com/opinions/a-prescription-for-baltimores-health/2015/05/22/582cbb4c-fa83-11e4-9030-b4732caefe81_story.html?utm_term=.8ca4d9afc0c4

Reflections on Engaging Public Health and the Larger Community

One person really can make a difference and there's no more important work to be done than in health.—Leana Wen

Wen's powerful stories point to a pattern in which the city's public health resources are used both to engage and rely on the whole community:

- Infant mortality has been reduced through a range of interventions that touch on the many factors that have an impact on a baby's chances of survival. Many practitioners and points of maternal contact were needed to make this happen, and will be needed to continue the progress so that babies grow up healthy and cycles of intergenerational poverty can be broken. It takes a community with a shared mission to break down siloes and chart the path forward.
- Potentially violent incidents have been defused by local people—individuals who may have been devalued by the larger community, but who turned out to be the right people for the job. Individuals from the communities they serve are often the most credible and impactful messengers.
- All Baltimore residents now can be lifesavers for people at risk of opioid overdose, a crucial first step in stemming the tide of the opioid crisis. Health is not just the duty of public health practitioners and health care workers; everyone can and should be involved in promoting health and saving lives.

Referencing Ta-Nehisi Coates, Wen underscored that "everything comes back to health. When you unravel, unwind everything, it always comes back to health." She emphasized the importance of bridging the needs that communities bring forward with the research expertise to figure out what will "make the biggest difference."

Measuring and Fostering Economic Well-Being: The Genuine Progress Indicator

To make genuine progress, we must be willing to adopt a more holistic definition of progress itself. To seek an honest assessment of whether our graphs are moving in the right direction—or in the wrong one. A system without feedback eventually fails. And our country, our states, our cities—they are all systems. Life creates the conditions that are conducive to life. Period. Full

stop. Perhaps, there is no better description of the intent of GPI. Its purpose
is to further the conditions that are conducive to life.—Martin O'Malley

In 2010, Maryland became the first state in the nation to adopt the use of the
Genuine Progress Indicator (GPI) as a measure of its economic well-being, an
example of creativity and initiative in government that pointed to an openness in
identifying and addressing key issues that affect the well-being of its residents. In
2012–13, the Center for Sustainable Economy[7] developed its first GPI analysis
for the City of Baltimore.

What is the GPI and How Did It Get Here?

After the 1944 Bretton Woods Agreement,[8] gross domestic product (GDP) was
generally adopted around the world as the standard measure of national economies. GDP is a measure of the monetary value of all finished goods and services produced within a nation's borders over a particular time period. Though
widely used, GDP has been criticized for a number of reasons including: not
accounting for black market, underground, or unpaid economic activity; being
biased toward manufacturing; and not capturing much that is valuable but not
tangible.

Growth is generally seen as being good for a country. To understand better
whether growth actually brings the things the country really needs, Lew Daly
and colleagues plotted U.S. GDP growth, which has doubled over the past
50 years, against several metrics. They found that growth has not delivered gains
in many important components of personal and national well-being:

- Personal income lags behind growth.
- The average number of hours worked per household has increased and people
  have less leisure time.
- Pension participation has decreased—growth has not made retirement more
  secure.
- Growth has not brought progress on poverty.
- Incarceration rates have increased.
- In the mid-1990s growth began to negatively impact "biocapacity," the
  ability of the planet to provide resources and absorb waste at a given level of
  consumption.

---

[7] The Center for Sustainable Economy (*www.sustainable-economy.org/*) is an environmental economics think tank working to further a sustainable society.

[8] The Bretton Woods Agreement established the international system for monetary and exchange
rate management.

- Income inequality has increased as GDP has risen—an indication that growth has been highly unequal. And health and social problems are worse in countries with greater inequality.

The GPI is a metric designed to better reflect a nation's well-being by considering factors not measured by the GDP. It includes 26 indicators and is always evolving, according to Daly. These indicators fall into three main categories: economic (e.g., income inequality, cost of underemployment), environmental (e.g., cost of air pollution, cost of net wetlands change), and social (e.g., value of household work, cost of crime, and value of higher education). In contrast to GDP, GPI has been mostly flat over the past 60 years, said Daly.

The State of Maryland adopted the GPI at the state level in 2010 during the administration of Governor Martin O'Malley.[9] Hawaii, Vermont, and Washington subsequently adopted it as well and other states have it under consideration.

Daly noted that political accountability over the past 50 years has generally focused on growth and employment. GPI introduces well-being into the equation and adjusts growth in relation to inequality. If a nation or state is growing in an unequal way, then dollars are being added at the top of the economic scale for those who do not need them for their well-being. If dollars are added at the bottom of the scale, utility is increased. So growing with equality is a greater level of growth than growing with inequality. As Daly admonishes, "Stop talking about how *much* you're growing. Talk about *how* you're growing. Are you growing in a way that promotes equity in the social determinants of health, for example? Are you growing in a way that's equitable? Then the standard of accountability is closing the gap between your output and your well-being."

Showing Results in Baltimore Through GPI Analysis

The Center for Sustainable Economy worked with the Baltimore Sustainability Commission and others to create a set of GPI accounts for the City of Baltimore using new methodology that allows for calculations at the local level. The Baltimore GPI considers three major factors:

- Economic benefits from consumption of goods and services
- Economic benefits from community and social resources, such as infrastructure, parks, and help from neighbors
- Hidden economic costs, like the social costs of homelessness, poverty, and crime.

[9] Martin O'Malley was governor of Maryland from January 17, 2007, to January 21, 2015.

The first analysis of the GPI for Baltimore, in 2012-13, showed a city on its way to economic recovery. Key findings:

- The benefits of household consumption of goods and services (about $14,000 per person) were greatly exceeded by the economic benefits from community and social resources (almost $26,000 per person). Of these, the economic contribution of unpaid labor—housework, caregiving, and volunteering— accounted for more than $8,000 per person, adding over $5 billion to the value of Baltimore's economy.

    Clearly Baltimore's economic well-being is more about the benefits of a high standard of living (leisure time, quality schools, parks, etc.) than consumption.
- Baltimore's GPI grew by 5 percent per capita between 2012 and 2013, re- flecting its economic recovery.
- The costs of inequality, underemployment, crime, and other social fac- tors came to $17,485 per person in 2013, limiting the growth in economic well-being.
- The GDP is not an accurate metric of economic performance. The Baltimore GPI per capita ($21,934) in 2013 was only 36 percent of the GDP per capita ($60,385). The remaining 64 percent was canceled out by social and environ- mental costs or spending (such as on health care) that is really a cost, not a benefit, of economic activity.

While there is obviously room for improvement, the results of the Baltimore GPI demonstrate the strength of the city's social and environmental foundation and its upward move to economic recovery. The GPI will be a useful tool to assist Baltimore as it moves forward with its plans for healing, renewal, and growth.

Reflections on GPI Research, Policy, and Practice

> *Not everything with a price has a positive value. And not everything with a positive value has a price.*—Lew Daly

The GPI is a way for governments to include well-being and equity in the measure- ment of their economies. Session participants raised several questions about its use:

What are the challenges associated with a larger uptake of the GPI among states and municipalities?

Perhaps the real importance of the GPI, said Daly, "is that it helps to change the conversation." There are limits to the GPI. It doesn't always mesh well with policy. It is a somewhat "clunky" grouping of "chunks of well-being that are actually very complex, multidimensional policy issues." But the GPI offers an advocacy lens through which to consider policies that begin to address well-being and equity. More precise measurement tools will be needed to drive policy development effectively.

Where are the biggest gaps in measurement?

There are significant gaps in measures related to the environment, said Daly, such as those that address issues like climate risk or ecosystem services.[10] "These are totally outside of our national accounting frameworks that guide monetary policy. I would point to climate metrics and the need to green our GDP as the big next leap forward."

Is there a broader framework that would assign non-monetary values where appropriate rather than putting everything in monetary terms?

The GPI takes a tactical approach in attempting to explain non-market goods (e.g., the value of volunteering) in monetary terms so it may be compared to GDP, with the hope that policymakers will pay more attention to them. But "deeper moral questions about what we value and how we should support those things that we value" are left to the side, Daly acknowledged, citing the example of creating carbon markets instead of regulating carbon production, with corrupted carbon markets (and not reduced carbon emissions) as the result.

How has the lay public been involved in the development of the GPI?

Economis ts developed the GPI and it is somewhat disconnected from public input, according to Daly. But since the GPI is more of an advocacy lens than a measurement tool, he suggested that community involvement is less important in shaping the model itself and more important for telling a story about a community and its needs. Maryland has an active GPI coalition that uses GPI to put a metrics framework around the story of community needs in the expectation that this framing will catch policymakers' attention.

How do differences in world-view affect the creation and use of the GPI?

Daly gave an example to illustrate the influence of world-view on the GPI. In Utah, conservation and community are especially strong values, so a good GPI

---

[10] The 2006 Millennium Ecosystem Assessment defines four categories of ecosystem services: provisioning (food, water, energy, etc.), regulating (climate and disease control, etc.), supporting (nutrient recycling, soil formation, etc.), and cultural (non-material benefits such as spiritual, educational, and recreational).

for that state signifies good ratings in those areas. Maryland, Vermont, and other states view GPI as a question of rights and of equity. These are "different world-views, but toward the same goal," said Daly.

What are the next steps and challenges for researchers and practitioners?

The GPI brings some sense of integration in that it is designed to replace a GDP measure already in widespread use. Yet, said Daly, there is a trade-off as "it doesn't have the precision that you need to actually shape policy development." Daly stressed that the many efforts to create a strong GDP alternative, or any framework to drive policy toward well-being, "still run up against the brick wall of politics." He continued, "The whole idea that better information is going to change policy is confounded by politics and . . . the self-interested aspects of politics, where well-being isn't necessarily what the people in power actually care about."

Leana Wen and Lew Daly both offered ways that governments can address inequities related to the social determinants of health. The practical interventions described by Wen strive to mitigate the negative effects of the circumstances in which many Baltimore residents are living their lives, while Daly offered a high-level tool for assessing well-being at a national, state, or local level.

Baltimore's challenges mirror those of many other urban areas. Its commitment to changing the dynamic by tackling some of its most intractable problems presents a hopeful look to the future. And implementation of the Genuine Progress Indicator by both Baltimore and Maryland is a real-world application of a broader metric. Both approaches offer models for other cities and states looking to reduce inequity in the social determinants of the health of their residents.

A Look Inside the Robert Wood Johnson Foundation

PRIYA GANDHI, MS, RESEARCH ASSOCIATE, RESEARCH-EVALUATION-
LEARNING, ROBERT WOOD JOHNSON FOUNDATION

BRIAN C. QUINN, PHD, ASSOCIATE VICE PRESIDENT, RESEARCH-
EVALUATION-LEARNING, ROBERT WOOD JOHNSON FOUNDATION

In her 2014 President's Message announcing a Culture of Health, Risa Lavizzo-Mourey, MD, MBA, asked, "What new bridges must our Foundation help build to make a Culture of Health part of the grander whole of what it means to be an American?"

With that question, RWJF embarked on an ambitious journey to "transform what it means to be a healthy nation." Along the way, we have been enriched by relationships with new individuals, organizations, and communities—many of whom may not have traditionally viewed themselves as important players in the health arena. In all of our work, we reach out to and collaborate with colleagues from other sectors who bring essential expertise and passion that complements our own. Some of these extraordinary people are contributors to this book.

In her Introduction to this volume, Lavizzo-Mourey puts forth RWJF's vision, Action Framework, and key strategies for achieving a Culture of Health. The chapters that follow illustrate how researchers, policymakers, and practitioners are joining forces and taking action to reduce inequity and to improve population health and well-being.

Since announcing our mission to build a Culture of Health, we have positioned RWJF to make large-scale investments in areas where we believe we can have significant impact. We know that no single sector can or should be "in charge of" creating a Culture of Health. This final chapter describes how we are working in traditional and new areas across diverse sectors to accelerate progress toward improved population health, well-being, and equity. Our programmatic work falls into four broad themes: *Healthy Children, Healthy Weight;*

Healthy Communities; Leadership for Better Health; and *Transforming Health and Health Care Systems.* The *Achieving Health Equity* team works across RWJF to see that the principle of ensuring that everyone has a fair shot at leading a long and healthy life is embedded in all of the work that we do. Our *Research-Evaluation-Learning* team threads through all programmatic areas to build a rigorous, transdisciplinary evidence base.

This chapter ends with a call to action to continue this work, to mobilize and harness the energy of people from all walks of life and all disciplines to "garner trust, galvanize support, and inspire others to help lift America to a level of health that a great nation deserves."

Healthy Children, Healthy Weight

> *Survey research suggests that Americans are ready for approaches that strengthen families with young children and that protect children most likely to experience trauma. To do that in a big way, we need more than science. We need a movement.* —Kristin Schubert

Much has been written about the importance and value of investments in the well-being of children and families. In *Fostering Healthier Environments for Children and Families,* Chapter 8 in this book, the contributors offer observations on policies that enhance or restrict the development of healthy children.

Kristin Schubert, MPH, managing director for the *Healthy Children, Healthy Weight*[1] theme, says, "Too many children lack access to healthy food, good education, stable housing, safe areas to play, and positive social and emotional environments. It does not have to be that way."

Through *Healthy Children, Healthy Weight*, RWJF supports a variety of studies and projects in social and emotional well-being, childhood obesity, early childhood development, and family and social support. A few examples of initiatives within this theme are:

A Series on Social and Emotional Learning[2] offers resources about social and emotional learning, and provides information for parents, schools, and others in supporting the healthy development of young people. A report of a 20-year retrospective study[3] in this series suggests that children in kindergarten who are more likely to demonstrate "social competence"—sharing,

---

[1] For more about the Foundation's focus areas, go to *www.rwjf.org.*

[2] *www.rwjf.org/en/library/collections/social-and-emotional-learning.html*

[3] *www.rwjf.org/en/library/research/2015/07/how-children-s-social-competence-impacts-their-well-being-in-adu.html*

cooperating, helping others—"may be more likely to attain higher education and well-paying jobs." Pennsylvania State University's Max Crowley, PhD, is one of the authors of this landmark study and a contributor to this volume.

Healthy Eating Research: Building Evidence to Prevent Childhood Obesity (*www. healthyeatingresearch.org*) supports research on policy and environmental strategies that have the greatest potential to promote healthy eating and healthy weight among children, especially among black, Latino, American Indian, and Asian/Pacific Islander children and children who live in low-income communities. One study, "The Impact of the First 1,000 Days on Childhood Obesity",[4] examined risk factors for childhood obesity from conception to delivery and from birth through age two. The study identified risk factors associated with later childhood overweight—higher maternal BMI and excess maternal weight gain during pregnancy; parental exposure to tobacco; high infant birthweight; and high infant weight gain. There are few effective early life interventions for childhood obesity.

A Learning Collaborative on Child Development, Education, and Equity[5] is an online learning network "that better integrates health care with child- and family-serving services and systems." The network aims to transform primary pediatric practice, provide opportunities for stakeholders to share ideas and support one another, and offer technical assistance to selected communities.

Healthy Communities

Some Americans enjoy environments that offer safe streets, adequate housing, good public transportation, nice parks, and access to healthy food, but too many Americans do not. RWJF's *Healthy Communities* theme aims to change that picture. Abbey Cofsky, MPH, managing director of this theme, says, "We support initiatives that enable communities and all of their residents to thrive and reach their greatest health potential. We help them to eliminate barriers to healthy choices and to build, sustain, and expand their capacity to promote health and well-being."

Healthy Communities is focused on creating the conditions that allow communities and their residents to reach their best possible health and well-being. This includes work that ranges across the social, economic, and environmental

---

[4] *www.healthyeatingresearch.org/research/first-1000-days*
[5] *www.rwjf.org/en/library/grants/2015/08/establishing-a-learning-collaborative-to-elevate-the-importance-.html*

determinants of health. Initiatives within the *Healthy Communities* theme
include:

> *County Health Rankings & Roadmaps* (*www.countyhealthrankings.org*) "com-
> pares the health of nearly all of the 3,000+ counties in the United States
> to others within its own state, and supports coalitions tackling the myriad
> social, economic and environmental influences on health." The rankings
> illuminate the ways living conditions affect health and the roadmaps pro-
> vide tools to help communities take action. They may also provide help-
> ful context for findings such as those of Princeton University's Anne Case,
> PhD, whose study of "diseases and deaths of despair" among middle-aged
> white Americans is described in Chapter 1 in this volume, *Fear and Despair:
> Consequences of Inequity*. Among the health ranking findings released in
> 2016, "Rural counties have had the highest rates of premature death for
> years, lagging far behind other counties. While urban counties continue to
> show improvement, premature death rates are worsening in rural counties."
> *The RWJF Culture of Health Prize*[6] "honors and elevates U.S. communities that
> are making great strides in their journey toward better health." The prize
> recognizes the unique ways that communities come together to solve their
> own problems as it also highlights common positive characteristics found
> across multiple communities. Louisville, Ky., was a 2016 prize winner.[7]
> Residents of the historically black Smoketown area of Louisville die nine
> years younger than residents of many other neighborhoods. Recognizing
> the inequity here, citizens mobilized to make Louisville a vibrant place for
> *everyone*. By working together and by turning data into tools, they realized
> some changes. Two of many cross-sectoral initiatives: 55,000 Degrees,
> which helps residents get higher degrees, and KentuckyOne Health, which
> provides preventive care to patients with high medical needs.
> *Invest Health* (*www.investhealth.org*) brings together diverse leaders from mid-
> sized U.S. cities across the nation to develop new strategies for increasing
> and leveraging private and public investments to accelerate improvements
> in neighborhoods facing the biggest barriers to better health. A collabora-
> tion between the RWJF and Reinvestment Fund, this initiative provides
> opportunities for 50 midsized cities to transform the way local leaders
> work together to create solution-driven and diverse partnerships. The part-
> nerships are focused on improving health and well-being in low-income
> neighborhoods by increasing access to quality jobs, affordable housing,
> and nutritious food, and reducing crime rates and environmental hazards.

[6] *www.rwjf.org/en/library/features/culture-of-health-prize.html*
[7] *www.rwjf.org/en/library/collections/coh-prize-winners/2016-winner-louisville-ky.html*

BUILD Health Challenge (*www.buildhealthchallenge.org*) is a national awards program that supports "bold, upstream, integrated, local, and data-driven" (BUILD) community health interventions in low-income, urban neighborhoods across the nation. By strengthening partnerships between local nonprofit organizations, hospitals and health systems, and local health departments, BUILD is focused on improving health and well-being in communities and spreading the learning broadly through national, local, and regional partners. The program is jointly funded by the Advisory Board Company, the de Beaumont Foundation, the Colorado Health Foundation, the Kresge Foundation, RWJF, and a growing list of national, state, and local partners who support centralized selection of communities, communications and PR, technical assistance, and evaluation and learning. Eighteen community partnerships became part of the BUILD Health Challenge in 2015.

Leadership for Better Health

Lasting change does not happen without strong leaders who have the vision, skill, and stamina to break through barriers and form resilient alliances to foster healthier, more equitable communities. These leaders work across sectors—in academic and government institutions, private corporations, and nonprofit agencies—and many have chosen careers in fields not traditionally considered part of health—transportation, children and family services, housing, or education. They hail from diverse rural and urban communities, varied economic and social backgrounds, and multiple racial and ethnic groups.

Achieving enduring change requires a critical mass of such leaders willing to depart from tradition to forge a re-envisioned and vibrant future. To that end, RWJF established four leadership development programs under this theme.[8] According to Pamela Dickson, MBA, associate vice president for program staff and managing director of the *Leadership for Better Health* theme at RWJF: "We recognize that creating lasting change and building a Culture of Health requires leadership from within health and far beyond. Through leadership development, collaboration, and funding for innovative projects, the programs will break down siloes and find outside-the-box solutions."

Through distinct but highly complementary areas of attention, the leadership programs promote the advancement of equity, the application of knowledge

[8] *www.rwjf.org/en/library/articles-and-news/2016/rwjf-leadership-programs.html*

in the real world, collaboration among individuals in health and health-related sectors, and attention to diversity and the needs of vulnerable and underserved populations. A carefully constructed menu of mentoring, annual meetings, and advanced leadership curricula supports the scholars throughout the program.

The programs are:

Culture of Health Leaders (*www.cultureofhealth-leaders.org*) helps people working both inside and outside of health—education, urban planning, technology, business, and other areas—to become effective change agents in complex situations and environments. They work in teams in their home communities to address health problems that persist across sectors. Leaders receive stipends for participation and funding support to implement a project.

Interdisciplinary Research Leaders (*www.interdisciplinaryresearch-leaders.org*) are teams of researchers and community leaders who bring health research to health policy in order to promote equity in their community. The program supports diverse cohorts of mid-career researchers and community members in a three-year fellowship. Funds provide stipends for a team of three fellows and they support a research project chosen by the team.

Health Policy Research Scholars (*www.healthpolicyresearch-scholars.org*) are doctoral students from disadvantaged backgrounds or groups historically absent from graduate programs. They may come from any discipline, but are enrolled in research programs and are interested in health policy. Scholars receive an annual stipend for up to four years and may compete for a one-time dissertation grant.

Clinical Scholars (*www.clinical-scholars.org*) are health care providers—nurses, physicians, pharmacists, physical therapists, dentists, and others—who work in teams to promote health equity in their communities. For three years, the teams work on projects to better connect health care with factors such as education, neighborhoods, and income, which have significant impact on health. Scholars receive an annual stipend to support their participation.

The Foundation has also continued its work in some existing leadership development programs. For example:

New Connections: Increasing Diversity of RWJF Programming (*www.rwjf-newconnections.org*) provides grants, networking opportunities, and skill-building supports to early and mid-career scholars who are "members of ethnic or racial minority or low-income communities and/or the first in their family to receive a college degree." *New Connections* also introduces the Foundation to researchers from underrepresented groups, whose perspectives on health and health care research can inform RWJF strategies.

The Summer Health Professions Education Program[9] is a "free six-week academic enrichment summer program to help qualified undergraduate students from minority and disadvantaged backgrounds compete successfully for health professions school admission, including medical, dental, nursing, and pharmacy schools." Host universities provide instruction in math and science, help with preparing presentations and building study skills, exposure to health policy issues, assistance in financial planning, and a clinical experience.

Leadership for Better Health also supports activities to involve the private sector in building a Culture of Health. From individual companies such as CVS, which has stopped selling cigarettes, to international bodies such as the World Economic Forum, which launched the Future of Healthy initiative[10] in 2015, the for-profit sector is joining efforts to improve the health of its workers, their families, and their communities. In our *Engaging Businesses for Health*[11] program, we support work that makes the business case for good health—identifying health indicators that influence the bottom line and illustrating how healthier employees increase productivity, for example.

Transforming Health and Health Care Systems

America spends more money than all other advanced nations on health care, yet we fare less well on key indicators of access to care, quality of care, and measures of a healthy life. For decades, we have watched health care costs escalate at alarming rates, siphoning valuable resources from urgent needs such as education, housing, and infrastructure development. The hardship is not shared equally among all Americans. People working in low-paying jobs, those with limitations in their ability to work, and people who cannot afford high premiums or deductibles are disproportionately affected.

The *Transforming Health and Health Care Systems* theme addresses topics including health care cost and value, health care quality, health coverage, and population health. Anne Weiss, MPP, serves as the theme's managing director.

[9] *www.rwjf.org/en/library/research/2011/08/summer-medical-and-dental-education-program.html*
[10] *www.forbes.com/sites/baininsights/2015/01/30/the-future-of-healthy/#1cc481db6e9e*
[11] *www.anr.rwjf.org/viewCfp.do?cfpId=1326&cfpOverviewId*

As she conceives of it, "To maximize the impact of our nation's investments in health and to achieve better health outcomes for everyone, we need systems that are more coordinated, that have the tools they need to promote better decisions, and that are better integrated with public health, social services, and beyond."

Some examples of initiatives supported by *Transforming Health and Health Care Systems* are:

The National Center to Improve Care for Complex Patients[12] at the Camden Coalition of Healthcare Providers is establishing a national center and up to four regional centers of excellence to advance the emerging field of complex care. The goal is to improve outcomes and reduce costs for patients whose complex medical and social needs drive them to extensive use of emergency departments and other costly forms of care. The center will operate an online learning community, organize technical assistance, and disseminate information about innovations and resources.

The National Health Security Preparedness Index (*www.nhspi.org*) integrates "measures from multiple sources and perspectives to offer a broad view of the health protections in place for the nation as a whole and for each U.S. state." It covers topics such as actions to monitor and detect health threats and actions regarding community planning for responding to disasters and emergencies. For the nation as a whole in 2015, "incident and information management" scored the highest, followed by "health security surveillance." "Health care delivery" scored the lowest, followed by "community planning and engagement."

Data Across Sectors for Health (DASH; *www.dashconnect.org*) "supports projects that improve health through multi-sector data sharing collaborations." By pointing to the challenges and opportunities in connecting data across sectors and by helping communities create and use data to inform change, DASH enhances community capacity to align health care, public health, and other systems that are essential ingredients of building a Culture of Health. With support from DASH, officials and academic researchers in Baltimore are using data to reduce the 55,000 annual falls among older adults through the Baltimore Falls Reduction Initiative Engaging Neighborhoods and Data.[13] City officials receive regular updates as to when and where falls are occurring, and data about other health, environmental, and social services factors that

---

[12] *www.rwjf.org/en/library/articles-and-news/2016/03/organizations-provide-8-7-million-to-launch-national-center.html*

[13] *www.dashconnect.org/2016/08/04/engaging-neighborhoods-to-use-data-for-fall-prevention/*

affect falls. For example, matching falls and housing data will help the housing authority address maintenance issues and provide information for a public campaign to prevent falls and reduce social isolation among older adults.

Evaluating High-Value Innovations from Low-Resource Communities[14] supports the evaluations of innovations undertaken in low-resource communities to improve health care quality and health outcomes without increasing costs. It also funds the dissemination of innovative strategies for potential use by other communities. Under this initiative, Houston's Angela House (*www.angelahouse.com*), a residence for women who are homeless or at high risk of becoming homeless, is testing and evaluating a program of providing holistic care to homeless women as a way of avoiding costlier incarceration.

Achieving Health Equity

Our commitment to achieving health equity and eliminating health disparities is both an agenda of work and a driving principle and philosophy that is central to everything we do. As Lavizzo-Mourey says in her Introduction, "Health equity means working together to make sure that we *all* have the basics to be healthy."

Achieving health equity requires working with colleagues across the public, nonprofit, and private sectors to change systems and policies that frequently restrict opportunities and limit choices to be healthy—unsafe housing, fragmented social services, struggling schools, mass incarceration, dangerous streets, and others.

Dwayne C. Proctor, PhD, RWJF director and senior adviser to the president, leads the Foundation's equity work. "Equity," he explains, "is the essential foundation for health and the hallmark of a just civil society. If people are not treated fairly and if our systems don't serve them well, inequities are inevitable and good health remains an elusive, unattainable goal."

The *Robert Wood Johnson Foundation Awards for Health Equity*[15] program "recognizes individuals within leading organizations that have successfully implemented systems-change approaches to achieve health equity." Winners of Health Equity awards include Youth Move National, the National Association of Free & Charitable Clinics, and others.

---

[14] *www.rwjf.org/en/library/programs-and-initiatives/I/innovations-in-value-from-low-resource-communities.html*

[15] *www.anr.rwjf.org/viewCfp.do?cfpId=1301&cfpOverviewId*

In another project, we are supporting the establishment of the Health, Opportunity, and Equity (HOPE) Index,[16] "a tool for assessing and analyzing the drivers of health and health disparities in multiple systems that control the social determinants of health: education, income, employment, physical and social environment, housing, safety, and access to quality health care."

Research-Evaluation-Learning

Achieving a Culture of Health will hinge on the use of sound, rigorous evidence that has been generated in concert with policymakers and practitioners across sectors, and has been effectively communicated to non-researcher audiences.

RWJF's *Research-Evaluation-Learning* unit spans programmatic areas. We know that we are going to have to build a rigorous evidence base to learn our way to a Culture of Health, which will involve gaining a deeper understanding of the problems we are facing, and a richer handle on the contextual and environmental factors that surround these problems.

The *Pursuing Knowledge with Purpose* section of this book provides some guidance in helping us develop that understanding. There, contributors offer insights about methods for generating and sharing evidence, and suggestions for ways to generate knowledge on behalf of a Culture of Health. Clearly, more attention needs to be paid to actionable ideas, to integrating health and non-health research agendas, and to understanding health and health equity across systems and populations.

After developing the Culture of Health Action Framework, we wanted to understand whether the action areas, measures, and dynamics we have posited make sense and reflect effective, collective action to improve health, well-being, and equity at a local level. To do so, we launched a *Sentinel Communities Study* (data will be available on *www.cultureofhealth.org*), which aims to understand the evolution of collective action for health in all of its variations and to identify new measures using sentinel surveillance. RWJF is tracking 30 communities to show how diverse regional, demographic, and community contexts shape their efforts to build a Culture of Health in their own ways, and the role that metrics can play in those efforts.

We established four national programs within the *Research-Evaluation-Learning* unit, allowing researchers to unleash their creativity and expertise to work across traditional boundaries, to focus on cross-cutting topics, and to attract interest from researchers who have not necessarily viewed themselves as

---

[16] *www.rwjf.org/en/library/grants/2015/06/creating-a-national-index-of-health-equity-to-assess-conditions-.html*

health researchers. All four programs solicit research proposals through open funding calls.

The research programs are:

Evidence for Action (*www.evidenceforaction.org*) supports investigator-initiated studies that will yield convincing evidence and findings regarding population health, well-being, and equity, and the impacts of specific policies, programs, and partnerships on those outcomes. Nancy Adler, PhD, the Lisa and John Pritzker Professor of Psychology at the University of California, San Francisco, serves as the national program office co-director. She notes that the program funds specific studies but casts a wide net in seeking ideas. Its solicitations do not limit topics that will be considered for funding, looking instead to researchers for ideas. A guiding question in weighing funding decisions is "Can the people who will use the research have enough faith in the findings to base decisions on the findings?" Adler says. In one study,[17] staff of the Seattle & King County Public Health Department and the Seattle Housing Authority are evaluating the health impacts of community redevelopment at Seattle's Yesler Terrace, a former public housing complex being redeveloped as a mixed-income community with housing, parks, transportation, and community services.

Health Data for Action is the newest program to launch and will make one or more highly valued but hard-to-obtain health data sets available to researchers. RWJF will serve as a conduit between data owners and researchers from academia, industry, and government agencies. Funding from the program will support researchers in conducting rigorous research aimed at producing actionable ideas to inform health care policy and promote a Culture of Health.

Policies for Action (*www.policiesforaction.org*) addresses how policies, laws, and regulations affect health. The goals are to promote policies that advance a community's priorities, highlight innovative collaborations, and foster stability and continuity at the community, state, and federal levels. Lisa Dubay, PhD, and Laudan Aron, MA, senior fellows at the Urban Institute, co-direct the national coordinating center. "Social determinants have enormous impact on health," says Dubay, "and policies and laws, in turn, have enormous impact on the social determinants." Sherry Glied, a contributor to this book and director of the P4A research hub at the New York University Wagner Graduate School of Public Service, is examining two

---

[17] *www.evidenceforaction.org/seattles-yesler-terrace-redevelopment-addressing-impact-multi-sector-strategies-redevelopment-plans*

kinds of housing policy. In one study, researchers are linking data on rehabilitated public housing developments in New York City with Medicaid data to determine whether Medicaid recipients living in rehabilitated housing have different health outcomes than recipients living in housing that was not renovated. Another study links foreclosure data to Medicaid data to compare the health of residents living in high-foreclosure blocks with the health of residents living elsewhere.

Systems for Action (*www.systemsforaction.org*) builds on advances in the field of systems research, directing attention to improving the capacity of systems to seamlessly deliver and finance care that will improve outcomes and reduce inequities. The program encourages inclusion of systems that do not view themselves as connected to health, according to national program office director Glen P. Mays, PhD, MPH, F. Douglas Scutchfield Endowed Professor in Health Services and Systems Research at the University of Kentucky. "We have to broaden our research lens to look at the larger constellation of systems that drive health, and then look at what we have to build to align delivery and financing across those systems," he says. Mays notes that the fragmentation, duplication, and variation in practice found within systems become magnified when systems overlap, interact, or fail to interact. One study is examining the process and impact of the implementation of a "Culture of Health" team in the Delaware Department of Probation. The multi-agency team works to address the health, addiction, mental illness, education, transportation, employment, and housing issues faced by people on probation in Delaware.

We also recognize that to build a Culture of Health, we need to learn from new ideas, places, and voices, leading us to value "outside-in" learning. Within *Research-Evaluation-Learning*, two teams focus on outside-in learning, which helps push us to think outside of our boxes and imagine a different future.

Global Ideas for U.S. Solutions: The *Global Ideas for U.S. Solutions* team, led by Karabi B. Acharya, ScD, MHS, provides funds to support the exploration and application of promising approaches from abroad that can contribute to a Culture of Health in this nation. Acharya explains its goals thusly: "While RWJF has always sought out new programs and strategies in the United States, we understand that we don't have all the answers here at home. So we seek to assimilate ideas from around the world and use that knowledge to improve health and well-being in the U.S." With support from *Global Ideas for U.S. Solutions*, we have supported the CDC's Division of Violence Prevention in testing the Cardiff [Wales] Model for Violence

Prevention in Atlanta and Philadelphia.[18] The CDC will fund community partnerships in each city to combine data on violence from police reports with de-identified hospital emergency department records. The combined data provide a basis for violence-prevention planning, action, and evaluation.

Pioneer: The *Pioneer* team seeks ideas that help take us into the future and offer us new and unconventional perspectives on building a Culture of Health. While remaining open-minded about specific topics or approaches, we find that many of the innovative ideas that appeal to us challenge assumptions or practices, put a new spin on an existing idea, suggest a new angle for an old problem, apply ideas from other fields, and examine ways that emerging trends can affect our ability to build a Culture of Health. Pioneer accepts brief proposals on a rolling basis. Lori Melichar, PhD, directs the program and explains its goals as follows: "With an equal eye to the present and the future, we aim to stay on the leading edge of discovery and spark a continual exchange of ideas that could help us all live healthier, happier, and longer." In one study, we consider that linking a person's electronic health records to data from his or her social media exchanges and searches might provide insights about factors that influence health, and guide medical providers in delivering care to patients. This project will collect data from 4,000 people, yielding lessons on creating data sets and on people's level of comfort with sharing these data.

We began our journey toward a Culture of Health back in 2014 and released our Action Framework in late 2015. The Framework is the compass guiding our work and, as Lavizzo-Mourey notes in her Introduction, invites "new participants by helping them see the transformative roles they can play, or may already be playing, to improve health for all."

With equity as our guiding principle we have deepened our commitment to children, made strategic investments in communities, promoted the development of new leaders, undertaken activities to transform health and health care systems, and strengthened our resolve to generate and share knowledge. These efforts have been further supported by our Communications department's strategic messaging and development of the Culture of Health website, among other activities.

---

[18] *www.rwjf.org/en/library/grants/2014/12/piloting-the-cardiff-model-for-violence-prevention-in-the-united.html* and *www.cdcfoundation.org/what/programs/list#program-1792*

We have learned that building a Culture of Health will require all of us to step out of our comfort zones, think big, and act together. We hope the Action Framework will catalyze action, with the understanding that we are all learning, adapting, and adjusting as we go.

In our 2016 President's Message, we issued a challenge to individuals and organizations to forge new and unconventional partnerships with the goal of building a Culture of Health that benefits everyone. We hope this snapshot of RWJF's current work underscores our intention to be part of that process.

PART SIX

CONCLUSION

ALONZO L. PLOUGH, PHD, MPH, MA, CHIEF SCIENCE OFFICER
AND VICE PRESIDENT, RESEARCH-EVALUATION-LEARNING,
ROBERT WOOD JOHNSON FOUNDATION

In embarking on our vision to build a national Culture of Health, we began with a central question: What is holding the nation back from the health status and heath equity to which we aspire? That led us to ask two additional questions: What do we know about that is evidence-based, but has not been taken to scale? And, what do we need to know more about to improve population health, well-being, and equity in this nation?

The robust discussions at and learnings from the *Sharing Knowledge to Build a Culture of Health* conference demonstrate that a vital national dialogue bolstered by innovative research and committed community efforts are necessary to inform future action. The chapters in this volume evidence the critical role that social determinants of health play, and how many drivers of change in these determinants fall outside of the traditional health care system. The cross-disciplinary research approaches and consideration of the range of influences, from family context to climate change, exemplify the type of inquiry that will strengthen the knowledge base required to operationalize RWJF's vision to build a Culture of Health.

RWJF is using the strategies and ideas presented in this volume to inspire our work as we continue to engage new and traditional partners and measure progress through our Action Framework. It is our hope that you readers, from different backgrounds and perspectives, will similarly leverage these cross-sector learnings to join forces and take action to build a national Culture of Health, for now and for generations to come.

BIBLIOGRAPHY

Chapter 1, Fear and Despair

Case A, Deaton A. "Morbidity and Mortality in Midlife Among White Non-Hispanic Americans in the 21st Century." *Proceedings of the National Academy of Sciences of the United States of America.* 2015;112(49):15078–15083. *www.pnas.org/content/112/49/15078.full.* (referenced on pages 12–14)

Chapter 2, From Disparity to Equity

Devine PG, Forscher PS, Austin AJ, Cox WTL. "Long-Term Reduction in Implicit Race Bias: A Prejudice Habit-Breaking Intervention." *Journal of Experimental Social Psychology.* 2012;48(6):1267–1278. doi:10.1016/j.jesp.2012.06.003. (referenced on page 25)

Lewis TT, Everson-Rose SA, Powell LH, Matthews KA, Brown C, Karavolos K, Sutton-Tyrrell K, Jacobs E, Wesley D. "Chronic Exposure to Everyday Discrimination and Coronary Artery Calcification in African-American Women: The SWAN Heart Study." *Psychosomatic Medicine.* 2006;68(3):362–368. (referenced on page 24)

Reskin B. "The Race Discrimination System." *Annual Review of Sociology.* 2012;38:17–35. doi:10.1146/annurev-soc-071811-145508. (referenced on page 26)

Chapter 3, How Americans Value Health

Bye L, Ghirardelli A, Fontes A. "Promoting Health Equity And Population Health: How Americans' Views Differ." *Health Affairs.* 2016;35(11):1982–1990. doi:10.1377/hlthaff.2016.0730. (referenced on pages 36–37)

Crum AJ, Corbin WR, Brownell KD, Salovey P. "Mind Over Milkshakes: Mindsets, Not Just Nutrients, Determine Ghrelin Response." *Health Psychology.* 2011;30(4):424–431. doi:10.1037/a0023467. (referenced on page 44)

Crum AJ, Langer EJ. "Mind-Set Matters: Exercise and the Placebo Effect." *Psychological Science.* 2007;18:165–171. (referenced on page 44)

Chapter 5, Measure the Change You Wish to See in the World

Gittelsohn J, Mui Y, Adam A, Lin S, Kharmats A, Igusa T, Lee BY. "Incorporating Systems Science Principles into the Development of Obesity Prevention Interventions: Principles, Benefits, and Challenges." *Current Obesity Reports.* 2015;4(2):174–181. doi:10.1007/s13679-015-0147-x. (referenced on pages 67–69)

Lee BY. "The One Thing to Do to Stop the Obesity Epidemic." *Forbes.* October 12, 2016. (referenced on pages 67–69)

Lee BY, Bartsch SM, Mui Y, Haidari LA, Spiker ML, Gittelsohn J. "A Systems Approach to Obesity." *Nutrition Reviews* (in press). (referenced on pages 67–69)

Wong MS, Nau C, Kharmats AY, Vedovato GM, Cheskin LJ, Gittelsohn J, Lee BY. "Using a Computational Model to Quantify the Potential Impact of Changing the Placement of Healthy Beverages in Stores as an Intervention to 'Nudge' Adolescent Behavior Choice." *BMC Public Health.* 2015;15:1284. doi:10.1186/s12889-015-2626-0. (referenced on pages 67–69)

Chapter 8, Fostering Healthier Environments for Children and Families

Jones DE, Greenberg M, Crowley M. "Early Social-Emotional Functioning and Public Health: The Relationship Between Kindergarten Social Competence and Future Wellness." *American Journal of Public Health.* 2015;105(11):2283–2290. (referenced on pages 102–104)

Chapter 11, Rethinking How We Police Communities

Brodeur, J-P. "*The Policing Web.*" (2010). New York, NY: Oxford University Press. (referenced on page 135)

Carpenter, JM, Gassner, L, Thomson, N. "Enhancing the Participation of Police as Collaborative Leaders in Responding to Complex Social and Public Health Issues in Australasia." *Policing.* 2016;10(1): 17–25. doi:10.1093/police/pav049 (referenced on page 140)

Geller A, Fagan J, Tyler TR, Link BG. "Aggressive Policing and the Mental Health of Young Urban Men." *American Journal of Public Health.* 2014;104(12): 2321–2327. (referenced on pages 136–137)

Kelling GL, Coles CM. *Fixing Broken Windows: Restoring Order and Reducing Crime in Our Communities.* New York: Free Press, 1996. (referenced on page 136)

Kubrin CE, Messner SF, Deanne G, McGeever K, Stucky TD. "Proactive Policing and Robbery Rates Across U.S. Cities." *Criminology.* 2010;48(1):57–97. (referenced on page 136)

LUMA Institite. *Innovating for People: Handbook of Human-Centered Design Methods.* 2012. (referenced on page 139)

Tyler TR. "Enhancing Police Legitimacy." *Annals of the American Academy of Political and Social Science.* Vol. 593, To Better Serve and Protect: Improving Police Practices. 2004, pp. 84–99. (referenced on page 141)

Tyler TR, Fagan J, Geller A. "Street Stops and Police Legitimacy: Teachable Moments in Young Urban Men's Legal Socialization." *Journal of Empirical Legal Studies.* 2014;11(4): 751–785. (referenced on pages 136–137)

Chapter 12, Climate Change Through a Health Lens

Ferry D. "Valley Fever Is Taking a Toll on California Prisoners—and It's the Government's Fault." *Grist.* Feb. 3, 2015. *www.grist.org/living/valley-fever-is-taking-a-toll-on-california-prisoners-and-its-the-governments-fault/.* (referenced on page 149)

Impacts of Climate Change on Human Health in the United States: A Scientific Assessment. The U.S. Global Change Research Program, Washington, DC. April 2016. *www.dx.doi.org/10.7930/J0R49NQX.* (referenced on page 145)

Plough AL. "The Impact of Climate Change on Health and Equity." The Robert Wood Johnson Culture of Health blog, June 22, 2016. *www.rwjf.org/en/culture-of-health/2016/06/what_does_climatech.html.* (referenced on pages 145–146)

Chapter 13, Public, Private, Nonprofit Partnership

Dear A, Helbitz A, Khare R, Lotan R, Newman J, Sims GC, Zaroulis A. "Social Impact Bonds: The Early Years." *Social Finance.* July 2016. *www.socialfinance.org/content/uploads/2016/07/SIBs-Early-Years_Social-Finance_2016_Final.pdf.* (referenced on page 159)

Chapter 14, Forward in Baltimore

Sarkar S, Wen LS. "Building a 21st-Century Health Department to Lead Baltimore's Culture Of Health." *Health Affairs* blog, September 20, 2016. *www.healthaffairs.org/blog/2016/09/26/building-a-21st-century-health-department-to-lead-baltimores-culture-of-health/*. (referenced on page 170)

Talberth J, Weisdorf M. "Economic Wellbeing in Baltimore: Results from the Genuine Progress Indicator, 2012 & 2013." Washington, D.C.: Center for Sustainable Economy, September 2014. *www.sustainable-economy.org/wp-content/uploads/2014/09/Baltimore-GPI-2012-2013.pdf*. (referenced on page 176)

Wen LS. "America's Public Health Crisis: Gun Violence." *Baltimore Sun.* July 1, 2016. *www.baltimoresun.com/news/opinion/oped/*. (referenced on page 172)

Wen LS, Lloyd MC. "Baltimore Is Attacking the Roots of Violence with Public Health Measures— and Saving Lives." *Scientific American.* November 1, 2016. *www.scientificamerican.com/article/baltimore-is-attacking-the-roots-of-violence-with-public-health-measures-mdash-and-saving-lives/*. (referenced on page 171)

INDEX